Felicitas Waldeck

Jin Shin Jyutsu

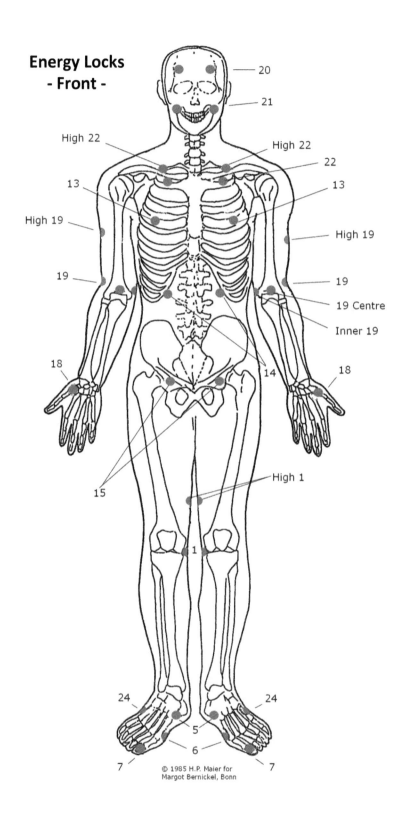

Energy Locks
- Front -

20

21

High 22

High 22

22

13

13

High 19

High 19

19

19

19 Centre

Inner 19

18

14

18

15

High 1

1

24

24

5

6

7

7

© 1985 H.P. Maier for
Margot Bernickel, Bonn

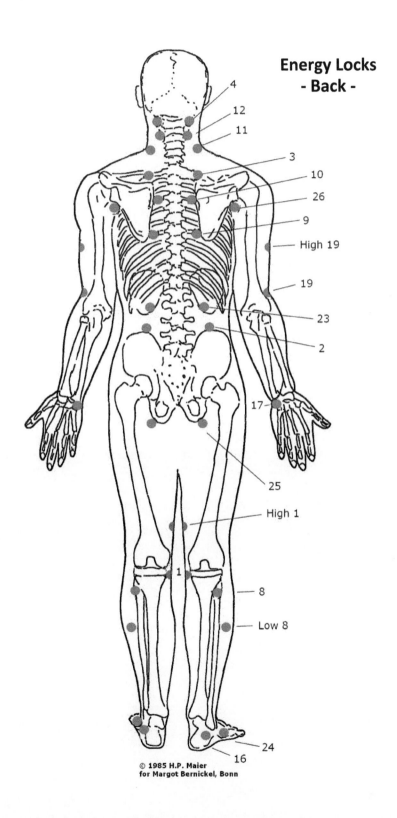

Energy Locks
- Back -

4
12
11
3
10
26
9
High 19
19
23
2
17
25
High 1
1
8
Low 8
24
16

© 1985 H.P. Maier
for Margot Bernickel, Bonn

Felicitas Waldeck

Jin Shin Jyutsu

Guide to Quick Aid and Healing from A – Z
Through the Laying on of Hands
No previous knowledge necessary
Immediate use on yourself and others

Jin Shin Jyutsu. Guide to Quick Aid and Healing from A-Z
Through the Laying on of Hands
by Felicitas Waldeck

Creative-Story
Safferlingstr. 5 / 134
D-80634 München (Munich), Germany
Tel.: +49 (0)89 / 12 11 14 66
Fax: +49 (0)89 / 12 11 14 68
Find us on the Web at: www.creative-story.com
Author's-Blog at: www.jinshinjyutsu.creative-story.de
Cover design and graphic digitalisation:
Creative Web Projects, München

ISBN: 978-3-942603-00-3
(Alternative formats and eBook versions of this title available.
For more information please visit: www.creative-story.com.)

Notice by the Author:
Since the complete organ flows have been published by third parties, I allow myself to present them in this book as well.

The drawings of the organ flows were created by Hans Peter Maier for Margot Bernickel (Heilpraktikerin, Bonn) in the year 1983. Both have given their permission to publish these drawings. The original illustrations are in his bequest in the keep of Susanne Wied, Berlin.

Notice of Liability:
The information contained in this book does not replace or substitute medical care. Anyone who thinks his symptoms may be serious belongs in the hands of professional medical care.

Table of Contents

The Knowledge is Already Within You

You may have always wanted to do something about your health but perhaps you did not know what, when and where to do it! Are fitness centres, jogging or cycling the right way or are gentler ways like yoga, the 'Five Tibetan Rites' or meditation the desired approach? Our brain likes to get challenged: for instance, travelling and communicating in other languages widens our mental horizon. The best would be a mix of everything for a healthy body, mind and spirit. Jin Shin Jyutsu offers this. Jin Shin Jyutsu literally means: *Human, Creator, Art*. Reading it backwards means:

The Art of the Creator through the Human Being.

When you start to practice Jin Shin Jyutsu you are on a journey of discovering the interrelations between your physical and spiritual self, which leads to self-knowledge and self-help:

The Art of the Creator becomes your personal Art of Life!

Initially Jin Shin Jyutsu appears to be new and strange, yet this knowledge has always been innate and just needs activation. For example while thinking intensely, you support your head with your hands. With this gesture you intuitively activate the brain waves, you are simply not aware of it. Nevertheless, you can easily awaken the potential of Jin Shin Jyutsu for your daily well being.

Mary Burmeister said: "*Be your own witness.*"

Start the first practice right away by putting your right hand over your left shoulder and your left hand in your left groin. Perceive how relaxed and free of tension your left shoulder is compared to the other shoulder.

This process of perceiving is Jin Shin Jyutsu.

I wish you joy and success in achieving improved health and balance.

Felicitas Waldeck

What is Jin Shin Jyutsu?

The Art of Jin Shin Jyutsu originated thousands of years ago. It harmonizes life energy by releasing blockages in the body. This innate art of healing is also called 'one of the Royal Paths' towards a mindful way of living.

The Japanese Master Jiro Murai researched and studied this old art at the beginning of the twentieth century. After his research, he revived and reintroduced this amazing art back to society. His student, Mary Burmeister, introduced this wisdom into the United States and her students then spread this knowledge all over the world.

Jin Shin Jyutsu harmonizes the energy of body, mind and spirit equally. This deep wisdom is innate in everyone's inner self and accessible to everyone through experience and practice. We do it intuitively all the time by putting our hands on the hurting body, be it the shoulder, the hip or any other part of the body. This way our hands serve as 'jumper cables' to support the energy flow.

Without thinking we expect that the body is able to absorb and process appropriately everything ingested and then to direct it to the corresponding body parts and organs. For example, a stomach medication is expected to be effective in the stomach only and nowhere else.

To delegate all entered substances, the body possesses an integrated circulation system of blood, lymph, nerves and messages to regulate and control the entire bodily functions, also known as the energy system.

Energy has many names and many slightly different meanings. Energy, however, is something essential, something vital and always omnipresent. All explanations of energy are incomplete and can only be an approximation. In Jin Shin Jyutsu, energy outside the body is indicated as universal or cosmic energy and within us, known as energy of life. The mediator between the outer and the inner energy is the central flow. This flow keeps us always connected with the universal energy and therefore our vitality.

The foundation of the Jin Shin Jyutsu knowledge are the 26 energy points also called 'Energy Locks' located throughout the body. There they develop their own vibration and have an important function within the complicated interconnection of body, mind and consciousness. While touching and holding these energy locks with our hands, we activate the energy flow and therefore induce harmony within us. Our body is comparable to a house with 26 rooms which can be opened with the Jin Shin Jyutsu keys. By doing this, these rooms are again put in order so that our soul can live in them and shine.

The easiest way to bring the energy flow into motion is to hold each finger individually with the other hand, because almost all energy channels move through the fingers and therefore can get harmonized. Children demonstrate this unintentionally by sucking their thumb which automatically influences the energy of the stomach, spleen and pancreas. Jin Shin Jyutsu is the art of self-knowledge and self-help; it keeps you in the flow of life.

To implement this art, we simply need:
- Our breath
- Our hands
- And the knowledge of the 26 energy locks.

Our hands touch gently two indicated body parts at the same time, even on top of the clothing. A noticeable connection is established when we perceive the energy as a pulsation in our finger tips. We have 26 energy locks on each side of the body. Their position and numbers correspond to the functions of the particular body parts (see p. 129 ff.).

Hands and fingers serve as a key to open these energy locks to make energy flow without hindrance. Now our body receives new impulses and energetic strength which activates the self-healing process. The energy locks receive their energy through the central flow that establishes our connection with the cosmos the same way the umbilical cord nourishes an embryo.

The conscious touch on the specific body parts is called 'streaming'. Hands or fingers touch lightly the indicated spots over our clothes without exercising much pressure. Being aware of the finger tips you will notice a rhythmic pulsation of the energy waves. The time of the application can vary depending on how pleasant and beneficial it feels. It is advisable to leave the hands / fingers on the spots chosen for at least two to three minutes. Hence it is important to aim for a relaxed posture.

For your daily improvement of harmony and energy we recommend:
- The 36 conscious breaths (see p. 19)
- The main central flow (see p. 20 f.)
- Holding all fingers individually (see p. 16 f., 64)

These three basic practices are recommended as a daily program for your energy momentum to be always optimally recharged.

In addition you practice the individual needed recommendations which are the:

- Finger practices
- Short versions
- References to organ flow
- References to individual energy locks.

Choose your own preferences that make you feel wholesome. 'Holding the fingers' is practiced while one hand holds the finger of the other hand. There are no restrictions, it can be done everywhere even with your gloves on.

Streaming / flowing can be applied any time. When you notice a change for the better, it will become a daily ritual. To make this 'holding the fingers' more understandable, the next page contains a detailed hand illustration of each finger with the related organs, its theme, energy locks and element. It is ideal to practice Jin Shin Jyutsu one hour each day. You can also divide this time in three twenty minute periods or two thirty minute periods.

An interruption in your practice, though regrettable, won't affect the energy flow.

A sequence of conscious touches is called a 'flow', better expressed as 'Energy–Function–Flow'.

The Hand

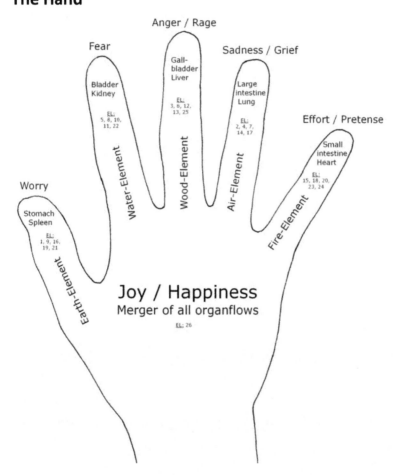

To choose the appropriate energy locks for certain symptoms, look at the individual key words in the chapter 'Symptoms from A – Z' (see p. 27 ff.). To practice the entire flow, follow the numbered hand positions row for row, either the left flow or the right. You cannot go wrong when you change the hands because everything in the body is connected. The indicated hand positions are just a selection of many possible combinations. If you cannot touch a mentioned body part for any reason, try to touch the same point on the other side or go to the next step.

When you practice Jin Shin Jyutsu on a daily basis, you contribute to your own wellness and happiness.

The Foundations of Jin Shin Jyutsu

The Breath

Mary Burmeister: *"In the Breath that I am, I am always renewed."*
The breath is our life's source and our ultimate healer. We can consciously lead our breath to certain body parts to activate the metabolism and therefore induce a change in our well being. But essentially we should be aware that we are oxygenated and that the breath is a gift to us.

Mary Burmeister: *"Our Inhalation is the Exhalation of the Universe and our Exhalation is the Inhalation of the Universe"*.

One of our daily practices therefore is our 36 conscious breaths. In just a few minutes we are replenished with new energy. With this practice we experience a deeper and lasting connection to the universe and to our inner source that provides us with all elements needed. We are part of the universe and made of the same matter. Our body is a miniature universe. Likewise only one drop of blood reflects a small mirror of the human being, as the human being is the mirror of the universe in his condensed energy.

36 Conscious Breaths

- Get comfortable
- Embrace yourself (big hug) while the hands rest in opposite arm pits with the thumbs on the chest.
- Get both feet grounded.
- Calm down as much as you can and keep your shoulders relaxed.

- Concentrate and be in your breath, let it come and go in its own rhythm.
- Breathe 36 conscious breaths and you will notice all your worries dissipate.
  Being aware of this practice helps get well again, because health starts in our consciousness.

The Central Flow

The main central flow is the connection between the universal and personal energy and when established, the filling station for all energy flows; descending at the front and ascending at the back of the body. Therefore it is essential to nurture the central flow with your hands daily. The descending energy at the front supports the exhaling and clears the head. Touching the individual body parts is crucial for the energy network and its supply. Each step in the following list shows you how to harmonize specific organs and body parts.

The procedure is as follows:

The fingertips of the right hand (R) remain gently on the centre of the head's crown.

The left hand (L) moves through the seven positions remaining on each one for at least two to three minutes. In the end you move the right hand from the crown to the coccyx while the left hand stays on the pubic bone. Feel now whether your head is lighter, your feet warmer or you experience noises in your intestines. Any reaction is welcome.

		Practice:	*Harmonizes:*
1.	R / L	on crown (middle of head) between eye brows	Brain function, memory, thoughts, sleep centre, sinus, eyes
2.	R / L	remains on head on nose bridge and tip of nose	nasal sinuses, eyes, urinary tract, reproductive organs, pelvic girdle
3.	R / L	remains on head right at the throat under the dimple	thyroid, adaption, metabolism, magnesium, calcium, supply, speech, hormones
4.	R / L	remains on head middle of chest	growth on every level, thymus gland, immune system, breathing, heart, soul's pain and injuries, guilt feelings, balance on each level.
5.	R / L	remains on head end of sternum	clears and strengthens the solar plexus, strengthens spleen and stomach, pancreas and kidneys, adrenal glands nervous system
6.	R / L	remains on head 2 cm above the navel	strengthens immune system in the intestines, protects our deepest soul layers

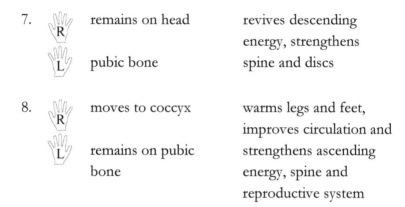

7.	R	remains on head	revives descending energy, strengthens
	L	pubic bone	spine and discs
8.	R	moves to coccyx	warms legs and feet, improves circulation and
	L	remains on pubic bone	strengthens ascending energy, spine and reproductive system

Supervising Flow

Beside the main central flow, to the right and left arises a supervising flow, taking care of each body half. In the same way as the main central flow they go down the front and up the back.

The supervising flows nourish all energy locks whereas the three energy locks (17, 18 and 19) are located in the mediating flow (see below, p. 23).

With two simple touches we can harmonize the supervising flow which influences our thinking.

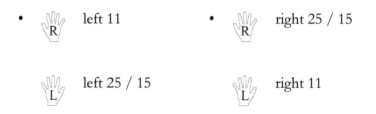

- R left 11
- R right 25 / 15

  L left 25 / 15   L right 11

Mediating Flow

The mediating flows combine both body sides and mediate from right to left and from left to right. That's why the mediating flow represents the acting principle, meaning it implements knowledge and benevolence in the two opposite sides of the body and combines them to one acting entity. Through solving old behaviour patterns, the mediator creates new solutions.

Fixed ideas and blocked emotions lead to attitudes that hinder us in our personal vibration.

Pythagoras (570 – 475 BC): *"Change your vibration and your life will change. That's how easy it is."*

The three energy locks 17, 18, 19, are located in the mediating flow on the arms. With our arms we embrace and show caring feelings, which change, nourish and activate a loving relationship.

- left 3

- make same ring

 make ring with thumb on ring finger nail

 right 3

put your knees together

knees together

Disease - What do You Want to Tell Me?

Mary Burmeister: *"Do not look at the name of the disease but direct your attention towards clearance of a blockage."*

Each disease is the body's answer of blocked energy and the weakest area reacts e.g. with a cold, with headaches or some other illness.

Instead of focusing on what is wrong, we should rather ask what is missing.

This question puts something in motion and does not manifest the disease. If something is missing, we move and look for reasons and go back to the initial changes of our health or the roots of our disease.

Slowly we begin to understand that a disease is the reaction of our body's missing balance, created through a lack of security, trust, acceptance and love. We understand that in our entirety the results of all our experiences are locked inside ourselves and remain stored. Hence, we do not want to get stuck with isolated symptoms, but rather consider the interrelations of the entire being.

For wilted house plants we immediately look for reasons e.g. brittle leaves, we check moisture, air and light conditions. Wilted plants are the answer to disharmony and imbalance in the environment. These symptoms are comparable to reactions of the human body to disturbances of the equilibrium.

Reasons:
- Thoughts become words
- Words become actions

- Actions become routine through repetition
- Routines lead us into a narrow corner and separate us from the abundance of life.

Unwittingly we create our own imbalances and blockages. The more we know about interrelations, the faster we can retain our health. Health starts in the consciousness. In recent years much has been said and written about consciousness. But what is consciousness and why is it that important? Consciousness is the knowledge of being and being is a condition we can only experience. The knowledge of being is studied in Jin Shin Jyutsu with our hands on our body.

My wish is to show you, according to your symptoms, a path of self-help which brings you into close contact and gives you a better understanding of yourself. You probably want an immediate solution for your symptoms, but without a deeper understanding, you will not achieve the desired results.

How to use the following self-aid instructions:

For instance for 'Lump in the throat' (see p. 84) you will find:
- a brief explanation,
- several instructions for fast self-aid (finger and hand positions),
- recommended organ flows,
- the energy lock: 14

Take your time, read the introductions carefully to find a suitable answer about possible influencing interrelations between the human being and influences like our seasons, climate, colours, emotions, etc.

Ask yourself the following questions:
- What body part is affected?
- Which energy lock corresponds to this body part?
- Which organ is affected?
- Which emotion is prevalent?

Always think: The body part with the symptom is the location of the least resistance. Perhaps its position can already give you information about the problem's interrelations. Practicing Jin Shin Jyutsu regularly will enhance your overall well being. Nevertheless, read thoroughly the meaning of the mentioned energy locks (see p. 129 ff.) to deal with your concern and thus remain healthier in the long run.

From the example 'lump in the throat' you discover the connection between 'liver, gall bladder' and a probable locked up rage. Via the organ flow (see p. 186 ff.) you will be able to remove this symptom. Practice the recommended steps daily and trust the effect to your entire well being. For every symptom there is a wide spectrum of possible solutions. Do not get overwhelmed by this abundance of possibilities but sense your personal concern and what your body wants to tell you.

Much joy and success be with you.

Symptoms from A – Z

In Practice and Application

The following chapter lists the symptoms from A – Z. Under each heading you will find a short description of related perceptions. You may recognize your current condition because your body may already be sending you a message of imbalance to your system.

Next come recommendations of which finger(s) to hold in order to influence the energy system.

The Jin Shin Jyutsu hand positions are indicated separately for each body side. Each flowing can be done on both sides. When you read, for instance R left 11, that means you place the right hand on the left energy lock 11 located on the left shoulder. Simultaneously, L left 15 means that you then place the left hand on the left energy lock 15, which is the groin. Keep the hands there as long as it feels good. If you have the desire and time, stream the opposite side as well. The corresponding energy locks for the opposite side are noted next to the first instructions.

Check the organ flows mentioned under 'To understand correlations' to find out more about the corresponding influences. As initially explained, it is not sufficient to care for symptoms only as they are a result of blocked energy. To identify the possible cause, it is important to continue reading the indicated organ flows in the chapter 'Organ Flows' (see p. 186 ff.).

At the end, the related energy locks provide you with additional explanations and guide you to the relevant chapter in 'The 26 Energy Locks and Their Meaning' (see p. 129 ff.). Each number corresponds to an energy lock not by coincidence, but has a precise definition and mission for each specified area.

When doing the individual steps you will notice an interdependence of numbers, symptoms and organs. This interdependence makes us one with the universe.

Acid-Base-Balance (pH Value)

The body's pH value and its role in health, attracts great attention these days.

The majority of western people are 'acidic', which roots notably in a mental instability we know as 'stress'. In addition, nourishment like white flour, convenience foods, including fast food increases acidosis as do addictions like sweets and alcohol. Since the symptoms have gone unrecognized for a long time, the aspect of acidity is overlooked unless a sudden reflux, e.g. heartburn, tells us something is wrong. You should take this as a definite sign that your body cannot balance acidity without your support any longer.

To harmonize:
- Place the thumb on the fingernail of the little finger

To understand correlations see:
- Organ flows: stomach, kidneys, bladder, gall bladder
- Energy lock: 14

Acne

The term 'acne' is a common name for skin conditions showing eruptions of red pimples containing pus, hardening, boils, etc., caused by an imbalance within the human being especially in puberty because of the hormones. However, this symptom can appear at any time in life.

The skin is our biggest secretion organ and simultaneously builds the connection between inside and outside the body. These visible skin reactions indicate a process of detoxification.

To harmonize:
- Hold ring finger
- Hold both 8

To understand correlations see:
- Organ flows: spleen, lung and colon
- Energy lock: 8

Addiction

Everyone is more or less searching and sometimes this leads to addiction.

One looks for harmony, for his purpose in life, for his potential, for his place here on earth and much more. On the path to self-knowledge, one thinks that one must define oneself through appreciation, respect, love, success power and knowledge. This path of continuing pressure easily leads into addiction, maybe alcoholism, drugs, work mania, gambling, anorexia or the need to show off. Each addiction is explainable by the individual circumstances.

It is not necessarily important to know the circumstances and reasons because these fixed behaviour patterns are being solved slowly when applying Jin Shin Jyutsu.

On this search one finds within oneself the hidden wisdom and encouragement to release new forces.

To harmonize:
- Hold both 23
- 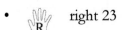 right 21
- 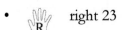 right 23

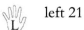 left 23   left 21

To understand correlations see:
- Organ flows: kidneys, bladder
- Energy lock: 23

Allergy

Allergy indicates a reaction to certain food, dust, pollen, chemicals, pet hair, insect stings and many more causes. An allergy pulls a trigger of an already existing disharmony of the body.

Jin Shin Jyutsu revives the energy flows. When blockages are opened, symptoms become weaker. Before allergies show up, previous blockages have been prevalent for quite a long time.

To harmonize:
- Hold ring finger and thumb individually
- Hold both 19
- Hold both 22

To understand correlations see:
- Organ flows: stomach, spleen, colon, lung
- Energy locks: 7, 9

Anger

What to do with anger when it affects you? Hold it in and swallow so it gets to us? Or do you release the anger on your family, friends and colleagues?

Anger divides soul and body, hence it is important to face the anger which makes handling it easier. Applying Jin Shin Jyutsu harmonizes and balances your sensations.

To harmonize:
- Hold middle finger
-     R   left 11   •   R   right 15

    L   left 15   L   right 11

To understand correlations see:
- Organ flows: gall bladder, liver
- Energy locks: 8, 11, 15

Anxiety

Anxiety is mostly not recognized as what it is for it has so many different appearances, such as jealousy, frustration, sadness and lack of fulfilment. A healthy anxiety-behaviour arises from being alert and therefore serves our security. Many people suffer from non definable anxiety.

Some anxieties are latent and their symptoms show up as bedwetting. Very deep-rooted anxieties can be experienced as depression or camouflage as workaholic behaviour. Nearly everybody knows a temporary anxiety, like during exams, correlates with frequent bathroom visits.

If an anxiety starts to strike you, try to find out where it might be located. Most of the time, it is located in the breast bone area or close to the heart or in the abdomen area. Place your hands on these areas and begin with the indicated recommendations.

To harmonize:
- Hold index finger
- Hold both 23

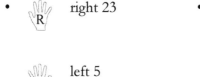 right 23   • 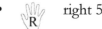 right 5

left 5    left 23

To understand correlations see:
- Organ flows: bladder, kidneys
- Energy locks: 5, 23

Arthritis -> see: Rheumatism

Asthma

Asthma is a breathing problem with pronounced difficulties while exhaling, caused by swollen mucous membranes resulting in coughing fits. The reasons are diverse and mostly originate in psychological imbalance and unsolved problems. In addition, environmental pollution is on the rise and is more and more an issue.

Be attentive and try to memorize what you have experienced prior to a fit of asthma.

Allergic reactions like fits of coughing can be triggered by pollen, viruses, bacteria, fungi and insect stings, to mention some of the possible reasons. By harmonizing your energy you boost your immune system.

To harmonize:
- Hold ring finger

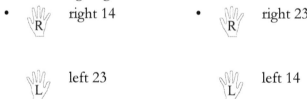

-    right 14
-    right 23

   left 23
   left 14

To understand correlations see:
- Organ flows: lung, spleen, liver
- Energy locks: 7, 14

Back Pain

Who does not know back pain? It appears in the upper back, in the lower back or both. The affected person looks for a new bed, gets a massage, or goes to gymnastics or swimming. All those measures can be very helpful provided it is the right bed and the correct swimming position.

The most important thing, however, is the right attitude. Be conscious of your breast bone and stick out your chest, and your back will automatically go into a straight position bringing relief.

Reflect on what depresses you, what weights are on your shoulders that make you look crooked and limp in your posture. Let your shoulders fall and *"be the falling of your shoulders"* (Mary Burmeister).

To harmonize:
- Hold index fingers

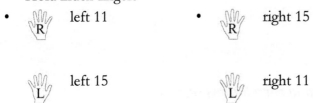

- left 11
- right 15

- left 15
- right 11

To understand correlations see:
- Organ flow: gall bladder
- Energy lock: 2

Balance

Jin Shin Jyutsu has three energy locks that concentrate especially on balance. EL 6 (static), EL 14 (lifestyle), EL 19 (mental state).

It does not mean that these three energy locks care exclusively about our balance. Furthermore the balance organ is located in the inner ear. Balance in all its aspects is depending on many factors. Each one of us can easily recall a period of balance loss.

We feel great and in harmony when in balance and all our energy locks are open to the energy flow.

To harmonize:

- Hold middle finger
- 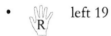 left 19
- 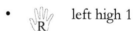 left high 1

  right high 1

  right 19

To understand correlations see:

- Organ flows: stomach, spleen
- Energy locks: 6, 14, 19
- See also: Dizziness

Bladder

The bladder function is related to the element of water, which is associated with fear. At the right and left of the spine the bladder flow has three paths on each side of the back. Fear makes the back muscles tense or even cramp, which can affect the bladder function. A weak bladder can also be related to kidney weakness or bladder irritation. In elderly persons a weak muscle structure often causes bladder irritations.

Pelvic training is especially beneficial. Remember to always keep the kidneys warm.

To harmonize:

- Hold index finger

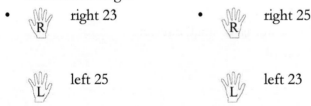

-    right 23
-    right 25

   left 25
   left 23

To understand correlations see:

- Organ flows: bladder, spleen, kidneys
- Energy locks: 14, 25

Bloating

Who does not know bloating, the feeling of fullness, which is particularly distressing when you have to remain seated at the table. If this feeling is the result of gluttony, then you can handle it relatively easily. If you frequently feel fullness after eating, you should seek expert advice. Select food and food combinations that are easily digested.

Hint: While sitting at the table, you can help yourself inconspicuously with Jin Shin Jyutsu.

To harmonize:
* Hold thumbs
* Hold both high 1 cross wise

To understand correlations see:
* Organ flows: stomach, small intestines
* Energy lock: 14

Blood Pressure

Hypertension and hypotension are treated equally by Jin Shin Jyutsu. The cause for both is mostly unknown whereas hypertension is prevalent. Somewhere in the arteries is a narrowing that causes the kidneys to raise the pressure to let blood pass through. Hence we need a kidney support.

To harmonize:
- Hold all fingers individually
- Hold both high 19

- right 23
- right 25

left 25
left 23

- left high 19

right high 1

To understand correlations see:
- Organ flows: kidneys, bladder
- Energy locks: 23, 10

Bones

The bones build the frame for our body. Though they appear rigid they are changing continually depending on the strain, posture, movement and nourishment. The stability is provided through our food, whereas calcium is especially important.

With aging, especially women face a change in their hormones after menopause. This lack of nourishment could lead to osteoporosis and susceptibility to bone fractures. Prevention is the key word and can be compensated for with proper nutrition (not too many milk products), movement in fresh air and practicing Jin Shin Jyutsu.

To harmonize:
*   Hold each finger individually

 right high 22
(touch beyond
the collar bone)

 right arm pit

To understand correlations see:
*   Organ flows: kidneys, bladder, small intestines
*   Energy locks: 2, 15

Cancer

The word cancer itself produces fear. The disease cancer is a holistic process and not a local illness. It indicates an imbalance of the inner milieu, depending on many different factors. Simply explained, the oxygen supply of the cells has changed, causing the metabolism going into fermentation. This can be the beginning of tumour growth. These bio chemical changes are highly influenced by our thoughts and attitudes. Hence we have to verify our old thought patterns, rethink and possibly initiate a change.

For each person facing cancer it is absolutely necessary to focus on healthy nutrition, exercise in fresh air and practice Jin Shin Jyutsu.

Read the individual organ passages to find out where the metabolic imbalances might have occurred: Sadness (lung, colon); worries (stomach, spleen); untreated aggression (liver, gall bladder); lack of happiness, joy of life, joie de vivre (heart, small intestines); or a collection of mental, materialistic things (bladder, kidneys).

To harmonize:

- Hold each finger individually
- left 11
- right 15 / 25

   left 15 / 25
   right 11

To understand correlations see:
- Energy locks: 5, 13, 14, 23

Cholesterol

Cholesterol the 'nightmare'! An elevated cholesterol level in the blood heightens the potential danger of atherosclerosis including an attack of the heart or head. This has initiated a wide discussion of the consumption of eggs and fat. So far nothing has been clarified with these allegations.

Cholesterol is supposedly a self-help product of the body to smooth out damaged vessels. Besides, there are different cholesterols, the good one called HDL = High Density Lipoprotein and the bad one called LDL = Low Density Lipoprotein, yet this also doesn't make it easier to understand the entire process. We know that stress, burden, hustle and genetic make-up can elevate cholesterol and that each person reacts differently to it.

To harmonize:
- Hold ring finger
- left 22
- right 23

 left 23   right 22

To understand correlations see:
- Organ flows: small intestine, kidneys
- Energy locks: 22, 23

Circulation

'I have poor circulation', what does this mean? What is poor or weak? Is it the heart, the arteries, the veins or something else? According to medical books, circulation is 'blood circulation' which includes the oxygen absorption in the lungs and the blood supply through the heart. Weak circulation or lack of blood supply creates tiredness, dizziness, fatigue or even fainting.

Jin Shin Jyutsu recommends: holding our wrists gives us strength.

To harmonize:
- Hold both hand wrists (17 and 18)
- Hold both 4

To understand correlations see:
- Organ flows: heart, kidneys
- Energy locks: 23, 25

Consciousness

In the last years much has been talked and written about consciousness. Many possibilities are offered to educate self-consciousness. But what is consciousness and why is it that important? Consciousness is the knowledge of being. Knowledge refers to studies where we need our intellect. And 'being' is a state, a condition, which we can only experience.

The knowledge of 'being' is studied in Jin Shin Jyutsu with our hands on our body.

Thus our understanding and consciousness will be awakened and experienced when practicing Jin Shin Jyutsu daily.

To harmonize:
- Hold all fingers individually
- Main central flow
- Big hug with 36 conscious breaths (see p. 19)

To understand correlations see:
- Organ flow: heart
- Energy lock: 20

Constipation -> see: Diarrhoea

Cough

Cough is a symptom with a variety of latent causes. If a cough doesn't go away there is cause for concern. A cough can indicate a weak heart caused by an energy blockage in the thorax. In general it is a symptom of a flu that has irritated the mucous membrane.

The lungs are an excretory organ. They detoxify the body through exhaling and coughing. In general it is important to support this function by drinking a lot of water and by practicing Jin Shin Jyutsu.

To harmonize:
- Hold ring fingers
- 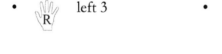 left 3   •   right 15

  left 15   right 3

To understand correlations see:
- Organ flows: lung, kidneys
- Energy lock: 22

Cough - Croup

Croup is a blockage of the throat and windpipe possibly caused by an inflammation and characterized by difficult breathing. Mostly affected are babies and toddlers.

First aid while waiting for the doctor:

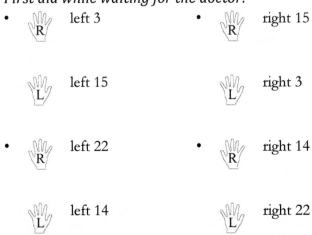

- left 3
- right 15

  left 15
  right 3

- left 22
- right 14

  left 14
  right 22

Dental Pain -> see: Teeth – Gums – Dental Pain

Depression

There are as numerous classifications of depression as there are as many processes of its development.

For the affected person it is very difficult to detect the right source of the depression. Therefore professional consulting is recommended.

Blocked energy and hormone imbalances lead to a reduced enjoyment of life and can trigger mood swings or melancholy or even a serious depression.

Long term depression may begin as sadness, sorrow and grief. As our busy lives demand, we don't allow these emotions into our conscious awareness.

Jin Shin Jyutsu describes this behaviour as an act of 'pretence', an attempt not to show one's personal feelings.

'Laughing outside, crying inside.'

With Jin Shin Jyutsu practices you strengthen and harmonize your feelings.

To harmonize:
- Hold all fingers individually
- Hold both 4
- Main central flow

To understand correlations see:
- Organ flows: kidneys, heart, stomach
- Energy locks: 21, 22, 15

Diabetes

Diabetes is a disease of the metabolism whereas the pancreas cannot produce enough insulin to utilize the sugar sufficiently. It is known that besides insulin medication, our diet is categorized in bread units. This needs to be watched carefully in order to avoid a low sugar level known as hypoglycaemia. Medical monitoring is crucial. Nurse practitioners and hospitals offer classes and guide lines for diabetics. Affected people have an ongoing temptation with 'sweets' in food and also sweetness in life. They normally demand too much from themselves.

To harmonize:
- Hold all fingers individually

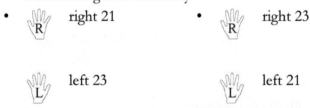

-    right 21
-    right 23

   left 23
   left 21

To understand correlations see:
- Organ flows: stomach, spleen, kidneys, gall bladder
- Energy locks: 23, 15

Diarrhoea

Diarrhoea and constipation are very unpleasant and can indicate something serious and therefore need to be clarified by a health professional.

Diarrhoea occurs for a short time e.g. while travelling. If the duration is longer, mineral loss needs to be compensated.

Constipation in general develops over a longer period of time. Laxatives are not a long term solution! The intestines get used to it and therefore an increased dose is needed.

Jin Shin Jyutsu activates the body's self-regulation system and distributes energy evenly and goal-oriented. We can trust our body - it knows what is good for it.

To harmonize diarrhoea:

- right 8

 left 2
(with the entire hand)

To harmonize constipation:

- right 2
(with the entire hand)

left 8

- right 3

left 8

To understand correlations see:
- Organ flows: spleen, gall bladder
- Energy lock: 8

Dizziness

Dizziness / vertigo is a disturbance of the equilibrium, peripherally or centrally. There may be various reasons: am I correct on my feet so that my spine is in the vertical position? Is the dizziness based on blood circulation? Is the cervical vertebra in the right position? Are the neck and / or shoulders tense?

The uncertainty caused by vertigo is considerable and can lead to depression. It is a great relief when the cause is detected. Very often no reason is found. Jin Shin Jyutsu can always help.

To harmonize:
- Hold index fingers

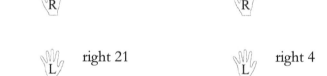

-    left 4
-    left 21

   right 21
   right 4

To understand correlations see:
- Organ flows: kidneys, bladder, gall bladder
- Energy locks: 4, 6, 10, 14, 21

Dyslexia

Dyslexia is usually an inherited impairment of reading and writing properly. Nevertheless, this can be compensated for with a variety of practices. Somewhere in the body is a blockage that results in this particular weakness. It is extremely important to practice Jin Shin Jyutsu for the entire body's energy circulation and to help both sides of the brain work together in harmony.

To harmonize:
- Hold both palms together (like praying) and draw a flat 8 in the air
- Hold both 8

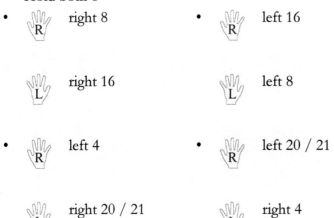

- right 8
- left 16

right 16

left 8

- left 4
- left 20 / 21

right 20 / 21

right 4

- left 3

- thumb on ring finger nail

 thumb on ring finger nail

 right 3

knees together

knees together

To understand correlations see:

- Organ flow: stomach
- Energy locks: 4, 16

Ears

The ear is our hearing organ and, the inner ear is the location of the equilibrium, or balance. Children often suffer from an inflammation of the middle ear whereas adults are more prone to a hearing loss including buzzing. For specialists including acupuncturists the ear is a map of the entire body. Earrings are gaining in popularity with both genders. Perhaps it is compensation for the constant annoyance of noise from headsets.

The ears have a lot of functions and there are many ways to help them.

To harmonize:
- Hold ring fingers
- Hold middle fingers

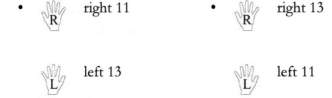

-     right 11   •   right 13

     left 13   left 11

To understand correlations see:
- Organ flows: kidneys, bladder, umbilicus, navel, small intestines
- Energy locks: 5, 6, 20

Edema -> see: Oedema - Edema

Endeavour - Effort

In our upbringing, much endeavour gets attention and is acknowledged as a rewarding guideline. This pattern follows us for the rest of our lives and makes us believe that only with effort we can be successful; be it with muscle strength, a strong character or appreciation and reputation. Would it not be great to achieve our goals more joyfully and effortlessly?

But primarily difficult circumstances aggravate the situation like misery, poverty, illness or other handicaps.

Jin Shin Jyutsu helps to find our balance and makes us strong.

To harmonize:
* Hold little finger

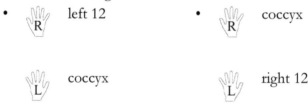

*   left 12   •   coccyx

     coccyx   right 12

To understand correlations see:
* Organ flows: heart, large intestine
* Energy locks: 12, 15, 19

Eyelid

Fascinating is the eyelid with its working ability as a shutter. As soon as the eyelid is closed, a completely different world develops in front of our inner eye. This little lid mechanism leads us from our 'realistic or actual world' into another dimension. Nevertheless, we are hindered by swollen, tired and trembling eyelids. Fortunately we can get help through Jin Shin Jyutsu.

To harmonize:

- Rub both palms of your hands and then put them on your eyelids

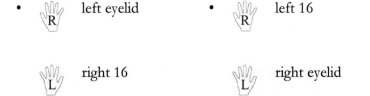

- left eyelid   • left 16

  right 16   right eyelid

To understand correlations see:

- Organ flows: liver, gall bladder, kidneys, diaphragm
- Energy lock: 20

Eyes

Sparkling eyes mirror a happy person; dull, tired or yellowish eyes make others think about one's well being. It is known that our eyes are the mirror of our internal life. Specialists, especially iris diagnosticians can recognize the condition of the individual organs of a patient by looking into their eyes. The eye is like a window that allows the pictures to go inside and lets the inside sparkle outside. Often blockages are located at a completely different body part and hinder a sufficient energy supply to the eyes. If the energy flow is optimized, the eyes grow stronger.

To harmonize:
- Hold middle finger
- 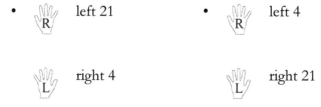 left 21
- left 4

right 4

right 21

To understand correlations see:
- Organ flows: liver, gall bladder, kidneys
- Energy locks: 4, 10, 20

Feeling Cold

One person feels good in short sleeves, the other person needs a warm water bottle and still feels cold. In general, it is a predisposition or constitution one takes without questioning. Looking at it more closely, we see a connection to the metabolism that depends on our food and its assimilation in the body. Consequently we are able to influence our thermal imbalances and energy.

A warm meal is suggested when feeling cold. When sweating, refreshing food is what the body likes. In addition we can improve the organ activity with Jin Shin Jyutsu.

To harmonize when feeling cold:
- Hold index finger

To understand correlations see:
- Organ flow: kidneys
- Energy lock: 23

To harmonize when sweating:
- Hold ring finger

To understand correlations see:
- Organ flow: lung
- Energy lock: 14

Feet

Foot reflexology is more recognized in recent years. It has become a general knowledge that the entire body is reflected in our feet. Jin Shin Jyutsu also knows these important energy locks in the foot (5, 6, 7, 16 and 24). In addition, feet and toes correspond with hands and fingers. A vacuum cleaner effect at the finger-toe-flow is created when holding the individual toes with the corresponding fingers (see: Finger). This is especially useful as a relief in an emergency.

To understand correlations see:
- Organ flows: bladder, kidneys, gall bladder
- Energy locks: 9, 15

Cold Feet:
- 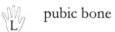   coccyx

  pubic bone

Fever – Temperature

Fever is an increased body temperature that is the result of an exceptional metabolic disorder. In most cases, fever is an unpleasant experience even though it is the self-help measure of the body to balance this disorder. Many people still reminisce of a compress around the leg dating from our childhood days. Jin Shin Jyutsu has a much easier way to reduce the fever.

To harmonize:
* One hand holds the opposite 3, the other hand creates a ring of each:
  Thumb and index finger
  Thumb and middle finger
  Thumb and ring finger
  Thumb and little finger
  When treating a partner, one holds the 3 and all fingers individually. If necessary both sides.

To understand correlations see:
* Organ flow: stomach
* Energy lock: 3

Finger

Our fingers represent our body's system with all its different levels and functions, but also serve as tools for practicing the art of Jin Shin Jyutsu. In general we place the three middle fingers of one hand on the corresponding body areas. In addition, we have significant finger-positions – called 'Mudras' - in Asia known for their harmonizing effects of body, mind and spirit. They can be seen in Buddha portrayals.

Master Jiro Murai practiced only the eight 'Finger-Mudras' for seven days and experienced a miraculous healing. He said to Mary Burmeister: *"One day you will experience the non-secret secret of the power that is in the consciousness and the understanding, manifested in thumb and fingers."*

This should encourage us to hold our fingers at any suitable moment, for our own well being.

Finger-Toe-Flow

People in critical situations or confronted with a sudden challenge can immediately get help with the finger-toe-flow:

Connection of:	right thumb	+	left little toe
	right index finger	+	left ring toe
	right middle finger	+	left middle toe
	right ring finger	+	left index toe
	right little finger	+	left big toe

For the other side connect the opposite points. It works like a drain cleaner.

Flu -> see: Influenza – Flu

Fungi

Is fungi infestation a fashionable diagnosis or a common disease? In any case, it is a phenomenon of our times. We see fungi on sick and dead trees; on them they disintegrate into flour and mix with the forest soil into humus. A similar conversion happens with the fungi on human toe nails or on other body regions in which they find a pleasant environment. Seen this way, we could call fungi our helpers to renew the damaged tissue. Sweets / desserts are a welcome food that encourages the growth of fungi. It requires an intensive work (fungi diet) to bid them farewell.

To harmonize:
*   Hold thumbs

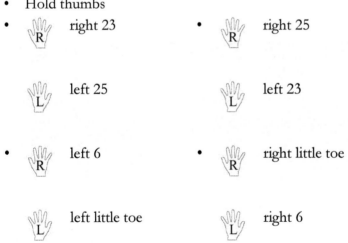

*   right 23
    left 25

*   left 6
    left little toe

*   right 25
    left 23

*   right little toe
    right 6

To understand correlations see:
- Organ flows: spleen, stomach
- Energy lock: 6

Gout

Gout is classified as a metabolic disease. The symptoms show up as joint pain related to deposits of uric acid. Elimination and production of it are not in balance. Drinking much water and practicing Jin Shin Jyutsu supports the process of flushing out the high acidic content.

To harmonize:
- Hold each finger individually
- Hold each toe
- Drink much water

To understand correlations see:
- Organ flows: kidneys, liver, gall bladder
- Energy locks: 15, 23

Grounding

Living here on earth means we have to come to terms with our surroundings. It is not always easy and many times it appears we have lost grounding and get lost in daydreaming.

In order to be aware of our inner balance we should practice Jin Shin Jyutsu daily. Only when we are in balance with ourselves, we are able to connect to the extreme ups and downs between heaven and earth.

To harmonize:
- Hold thumb
- Hold both 14 crosswise
- Self embracement (big hug), 36 conscious breaths

To understand correlations see:
- Main central flow
- Organ flows: stomach, spleen
- Energy locks: 6, 7, 1

Guilt

Many people carry guilt around with them which is not properly defined. Just as indefinable is their state of health. Perhaps an angina is noticeable, severe respiratory difficulties, menstrual disorder, low vitality or even addictions. A feeling of guilt can be treated through certain steps such as open conversations, a clarification or an apology for the behaviour that created the guilty feelings. In addition, we can work on ourselves, for example with meditation, contemplation or prayer. Jin Shin Jyutsu can especially be helpful because it stabilizes and helps us get to know our selves.

To harmonize:
- Hold ring fingers
- Hold both 13 cross wise

To understand correlations see:
- Organ flows: lungs, kidneys
- Energy lock: 13

Gums -> see: Teeth – Gums – Dental Pain

Gynaecological Disorder

The monthly cycle exists therein that a nest is built in the uterus waiting for a fertilized egg. A discharged egg is experienced in the monthly period. Much energy is needed for this process. If this area lacks energy, cramps and other pains will be experienced. Scars can also trigger those troubles.

Menopause indicates a hormonal decrease in a woman's cycle.

The central flow compensates and supplies the uterus with the needed energy.

To harmonize:
- Main central flow
- Hold both 13
- right sacrum
- right high 1

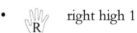 left high 1

left sacrum

To understand correlations see:
- Organ flows: spleen, kidneys
- Energy lock: 13

Hands

Quotation of Mary Burmeister: *"The Creator has at the end of His arms only our hands."*

In our hands is a particular energy and with them, we can treat ourselves and others. The hands have the ability to give new impulses like consoling, holding, easing pain, giving comfort, warmth and security. All this is general knowledge passed down through generations. However, did you know that they are not only our tools but that the entire body and its functions are represented in our hands?

With our hands we can harmonize the entire body. By placing them on the body, a sudden start is initiated which puts energy in motion.

The palms of our hands relate to our centre. To touch them as in prayer is the short form of the main central flow. When we clap our hands, like after a concert, we are led to our centre that grounds us.

Hands – cold

Cold hands and feet are not pleasant and more prevalent amongst women than men.

This is related to the metabolism whereas the appropriate diet can initiate an effective boost. Too much dairy and fat slow the metabolism down and too much raw food and citrus fruits cools it. These foods are especially chosen by women in the assumption it will help them slim down. The opposite is mostly the case because our body needs more energy to burn and utilize the food. Hence this energy then is missing to balance the appropriate body temperature. Fat deposits in the body are the visible results of this procedure.

To harmonize:
- 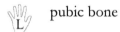 coccyx

  pubic bone

- right 25

  left 25

To understand correlations see:
- Organ flows: kidneys, bladder gall bladder
- Energy locks: 9, 11, 15

Hay Fever -> see: Allergy

Headaches

Headaches are experienced and known by the population in the entire world. They are not only symptoms of an illness but also a bodily reaction to fatigue, stress, insufficient nutrition and changes in the weather. If they are not only remnants of long partying and no change is noticeable, we have to look for the real cause.

To harmonize:
- Hold each finger individually

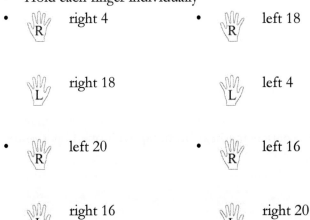

-     right 4   •   left 18

    right 18   left 4

-     left 20   •   left 16

    right 16   right 20

To understand correlations see:
- Organ flows: stomach, gall bladder, bladder
- Energy locks: 6, 16

Heartburn

In general many people seem to accept heartburn as a natural state of health. But heartburn always has a reference to a local or general acidosis, which requires attention. Diet should carefully be observed. If a person is troubled by frequent occurrences of heartburn, medical treatment must be obtained. Until then get help with Jin Shin Jyutsu-practices.

To harmonize:
- Hold thumbs
- Place thumb on little finger

To understand correlations see:
- Organ flows: stomach, gall bladder, bladder
- Energy lock: 14

Hint: When experiencing heartburn, tap with one finger onto the upper lip.

Herpes

As commonly known, herpes is very unpleasant, painful and contagious. Whenever the immune system is weakened the herpes virus recurs. This can happen when a person is physically challenged or when a psychological-mental tension is prevalent as in taking exams or going to one's wedding.

Herpes does not only affect the lips but can also show up on other mucous membranes.

Especially painful and serious is another herpes form known as shingles. In this case immediate medical attention is recommended.

To harmonize:

- Hold thumbs
- Hold both 8
-   on the herpes
     (not touching)

     22 area - vertical below

To understand correlations see:

- Organ flows: spleen, stomach
- Energy lock: 8

Hiccup

Hiccup is a term for involuntary contractions of the diaphragm, audible in a gasping breathing. Almost everyone knows that from personal experience. It can be very tiring, but usually ends fast.

It once affected a pope who suffered for weeks from hiccups. The Vatican searched the entire world for experts to bring him immediate relief with no success. A pity Jin Shin Jyutsu was not yet as widespread as today.

To harmonize:
- Hold both high 1 cross wise
- Hold both 12
- Hold both 14 cross wise

-     left 14
-     left 19

    right 19   right 14

To understand correlations see:
- Organ flow: spleen
- Energy locks: 1, 14

Hyperactive Children

It is an unpleasant situation for affected children as well as for their parents. There are many self-help organizations which provide a pool of shared experiences.

Primarily, the metabolism is too speedy, which we slow down by food prepared with good oils and thick butter on bread. In addition Jin Shin Jyutsu is an option that can further help to harmonize this imbalanced energy. The children will benefit from a newly regulated energy.

To harmonize:

- right 23
- right 25

  left 25
  left 23

- right 4
- right 21

  left 21
  left 4

To understand correlations see:

- Organ flows: stomach, spleen
- Energy locks: 23, 25

Influenza – Flu

Almost everything related to headache, cough and sore throat is called influenza. A real flu is a virus infection, weakens the body tremendously and can even lead to lasting impairments. Therefore it is necessary to be careful. Each one of us has experienced the flu and has chosen his own treatment such as a sauna, hot bath or his warm bed and sipping some special hot concoction. Consulting a physician should also be strongly considered.

However, remember to practice Jin Shin Jyutsu.

To harmonize:
- Hold each finger individually
- One hand holds the 3 on the opposite side, the other hand creates a ring of each of the following finger pairs:
  thumb and index finger
  thumb and middle finger
  thumb and ring finger
  thumb and little finger

Insomnia - Relaxation

Who does not know 'counting sheep' when lying in bed, again and again turning over, tossing around, looking at the clock and counting the hours until it's time to get up.

Sleep holds body and soul together – the saying goes, however, each individual needs a different quantity of sleep in order to feel comfortable. Meditating people train to sleep less, Jin Shin Jyutsu people need less sleep via streaming, therefore faster and faster the day's events say good bye and you plunge into your desired sleep.

To harmonize:
- Hold each finger individually
- Hold both 18

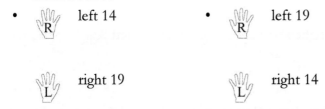

- left 14
- left 19

- right 19
- right 14

To understand correlations see:
- Organ flows: stomach, umbilicus
- Energy locks: 4, 17, 18

Knee

Many people have knee problems. Why does this happen?
The knee is the carrier of a heavy load, is very stable but at the same time very sensitive. According to Jin Shin Jyutsu-understanding, most of the energy passes through the knee, reflecting blockages of other body parts. For example: a tennis-elbow can also be connected to a painful knee. This again demonstrates that we have to look at pain in its entirety.

To harmonize:
- Hold thumbs
- Hold both 1, hands crossed

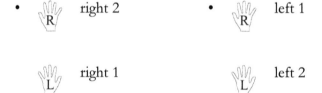

- right 2
- left 1

right 1

left 2

To understand correlations see:
- Organ flow: stomach
- Energy locks: 1, 10, 15

Legs – Heavy and Swollen

We already know that the nourishing vital energy flows down the front and up the back. Swollen, heavy legs indicate that this energy circulation is blocked. Other indicators are also prominent veins, weak connective tissue, hip imbalances and many more critical issues that should be checked by a health professional.

To get reenergized, walking outside or sportive activities in fresh air are very helpful.

To harmonize:

- Hold both hips with your hands (2)

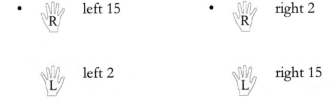

R — left 15	R — right 2
L — left 2	L — right 15

To understand correlations see:

- Organ flows: gall bladder, kidneys
- Energy locks: 2, 15

Love–Life

Love-life is a significant part of life's love namely the lust and joy of life. Love is an event in its entirety and not a local mission though one might think differently. Love is experienced individually - as seconds or a minute phenomenon – but it still influences the entire being. Love inspires, enhances creativity and releases strength. When love takes possession of body, mind and soul, the capability of love is developed and gets unfolded. Love now can emanate from the heart and inspire people in their entire life. 'Love Birds' are hardly ever sick because they are in the flow of their energy.

According to Asian understanding 'heart-love' gets nourished through the energy of our kidneys, they bring a certain contingent of love-power with them. Therefore, it is very important that kidneys are properly nourished, nursed and strengthened.

To harmonize:
• Hold both palms
• Hold both 13

To understand correlations see:
• Organ flows: kidneys, stomach, spleen
• Energy lock: 13

Lumbago

Lumbago strikes suddenly, mostly in the loin area, but can as well radiate into the upper spine.

Also very painful is sciatica which influences life quality tremendously. Pain from pressure on the sciatic nerve can radiate as far as the toes. Since the muscular system is tense, the body compensates by adopting a one-sided posture which makes the situation even worse. Lumbago is often triggered by physical and psychological challenges.

To harmonize:

- Hold index fingers

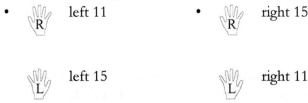

-     left 11   •   right 15

    left 15   right 11

To understand correlations see:

- Organ flow: bladder
- Energy locks: 11, 12

Lump in the Throat

The medical term for a 'lump in the throat' is 'globus hystericus'. In the medical handbook it is referred to as 'globus feeling', also a probable physical manifestation of certain emotional conditions. Emphasized is that no connection to a psychological disease is established. But this is often the hypothesis for its relation to the term 'globus hystericus'. This leads to a connection to the uterus (uterus = hystericus).

A 'globus feeling' therefore should not simply be categorized as 'hysteria' but taken seriously as manifested and locked in feelings. It could be a blocked rage not properly dealt with that should be harmonized.

To harmonize:
- Hold middle fingers
- 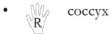 coccyx
- 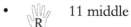 11 middle

 11 middle

 coccyx

To understand correlations see:
- Organ flows: liver, gall bladder
- Energy lock: 14
- See also: Neck - Throat

Lymph

Lymph is a pale, yellow liquid that flows in the tissue of the body, depending on blood and muscle pressure. In its pathways are lymph nodes in which the lymph is purified before it flows back into the blood circulation. Since muscle motion stimulates the lymph flow, we should move in fresh air and breathe consciously.

To harmonize:
- Hold each finger individually

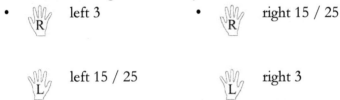

-      left 3   •   right 15 / 25

     left 15 / 25   right 3

To understand correlations see:
- Organ flows: spleen, stomach
- Energy locks: 3, 15

Metabolism

Metabolism refers to all processes in the body: from the absorption (of food, oxygen, etc.), through conversion, to excretion. Decomposition and reconstruction of body elements are also part of the metabolism.

People are generally born with a fast metabolism, which slows down throughout life. Women are especially affected by the reduction of their metabolic rate.

The simple maintenance of the individual and complicated metabolism requires a lot of energy which must be renewed continuously. Energy is renewed through eating, drinking, recreation and Jin Shin Jyutsu.

To harmonize:
- Hold each finger individually
- Main central flow
- Self embracement (big hug) and 36 conscious breaths

To understand correlations see:
- Organ flows: small intestines, kidneys
- Energy lock: 13

Migraine

Migraine is a very specific type of headache usually affecting only one side of the head that can be accompanied by nausea, vomiting, dizziness and sensitivity to light. In many instances migraine is closely connected to menstruation and emotions like annoyance, jealousy, rivalry and fear. Usually standard pain relief medications are only marginally effective for migraines because the blood flow in the arteries is blocked by partial spasms.

Many people suffer silently with migraine attacks. We suggest to immediately start practicing Jin Shin Jyutsu to bring the suffering to an end.

To harmonize:
- Hold middle fingers

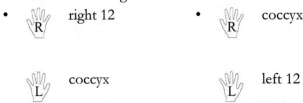

- 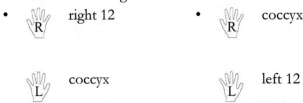 right 12
- 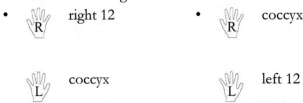 coccyx

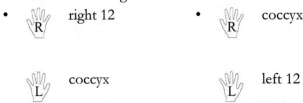 coccyx   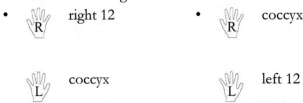 left 12

To understand correlations see:
- Organ flows: gall bladder, stomach, bladder
- Energy locks: 4, 14, 16

Mind

The philosophy of Jin Shin Jyutsu demonstrates the connection between mind and physical levels. Attitudes and actions build the structure of our body's tissue. In other words, the mind builds and forms the body. This also means that with our thoughts and consciousness we can influence and shape our physical body.

The energy follows immediately where our consciousness leads it. Therefore it is very important to develop our awareness and experience a feeling of well being while practicing Jin Shin Jyutsu daily.

Other therapies also sustain this development with specific breathing, visualization exercises, e.g. Qi Gong, Tai Chi, and others. Heartfelt meditation and prayer are an important support. Using our hands, Jin Shin Jyutsu easily leads us to reach the right inner attitude.

To harmonize:
- Self embracement (big hug), 36 conscious breaths
- Main central flow
- Hold all fingers individually

Movement

Movement has become popular and is of great significance. It is not only related to physical movement but also to 'internal movements' of the body, called energy flow. If the energy flow is blocked, one's complete life essence, such as blood and lymph flow, stagnates. Disharmony occurs because the organs are inefficiently supplied which makes one feel sick.

Through consciously breathing, positive thoughts and feelings and through practicing Jin Shin Jyutsu it is possible to keep and promote our energy flow.

Sports and exercising is an important factor and is recommended on a daily basis. It can be Yoga, Tai Chi, Qi Gong, walking, bicycling, swimming and many more activities.

But it is also important that exercise and movement should be joyful. Physical force without sufficient oxygen can lead to acidity and this can cause bodily harm.

To harmonize:
- Thumb on ring-finger-nail (for more oxygen)
- Hold both 25

To understand correlations see:
- Organ flows: lung, kidneys
- Energy lock: 25

Muscles

Showing off muscles is in! Muscles are the meaty part of the body with the ability of contractions. That's why they can be trained easily. If a muscle is trained, over-trained or torn, we experience muscle pain but the body can also respond with pain when a tense muscle has been relaxed, for example with Jin Shin Jyutsu. As the energy flow nourishes the muscle well it becomes soft, permeable and yet strong. Jin Shin Jyutsu makes muscles and joints flexible and builds them up without adding bulk like 'Mr. Muscleman'.

To harmonize:
- Hold index fingers

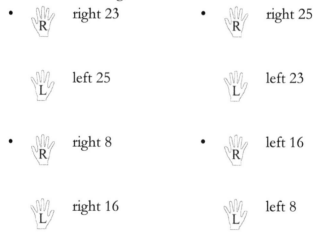

- right 23
- left 25
- right 25
- left 23

- right 8
- right 16
- left 16
- left 8

To understand correlations see:
- Organ flows: spleen, liver, bladder
- Energy locks: 8, 16

Nails

Fingernails, toenails and hair can tell many stories about us, but we are usually not aware of these messages: for instance when nails are brittle, have spots or show lines or when hair falls out, becomes dull and thinner. In many cases fatigue or great effort are the reasons. Insufficient minerals can be the cause but before replacing any of them, we should get harmonized through Jin Shin Jyutsu.

To harmonize:
• Hold each finger individually
• Hold both 22 cross wise, also effective against losing hair

To understand correlations see:
• Organ flows: kidneys, spleen, stomach, liver, small intestines
• Energy locks: 22, 23

Nasal Cavity

The head has many cavities: nose, jaws, forehead, and so on. All are filled with air and lined on the inside with mucous membrane allowing bacteria and viruses to settle down in this comfortable moist environment. Therefore it is very hard to get rid of them. These cavities need, at any rate, to be freed from those unwelcome settlers with Jin Shin Jyutsu. For those who can stand it, a saline rinse is very helpful.

To harmonize:
- Hold ring fingers
- Hold both 4
- 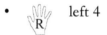 left 4

- 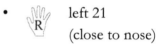 left 21
  (close to nose)

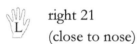 right 21
(close to nose)

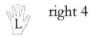 right 4

To understand correlations see:
- Organ flows: lungs, colon, bladder
- Energy locks: 4, 9

Neck - Throat

Some 'have a thick neck' or make 'a long neck', some have a 'frog in the throat' or they simply 'break their neck'. Those standard quotations make us aware of how important this body part is. First we swallow pleasant and unpleasant situations and later unprocessed feelings and emotions will surface again to be transformed by our consciousness. Vessels, nerves and energy supplying the shoulders, arms, hands and fingers, pass through the neck. Check your own neck and head posture if any symptoms arise in this region e.g. loss of voice.

To harmonize:
* Hold middle finger
*   left 12

    coccyx

*   left 3

    left 15, 25

*   coccyx

    right 12

*   right 15, 25

    right 3

To understand correlations see:
- Organ flows: bladder, liver, stomach
- Energy locks: 3, 10, 11, 12

Nerves

In earlier times we had one 'nerve doctor' who took care of the nerves on the physical level as well as on the psychological.

Today we have an increasing specialization. In this context, the different levels are characterized by the word 'psychosomatic' (soma = body). Usually we are not aware that a disease may have a psychological origin. A person who is in a state of nervous exhaustion must be energetically nourished, for example with joy and laughter, with good food and of course with Jin Shin Jyutsu.

The creation of the nerves belongs to our basis and to the element earth (spleen). When the nerves 'explode', they are then associated with the fire element (small intestines).

To harmonize:
- Hold thumbs
- Hold little fingers

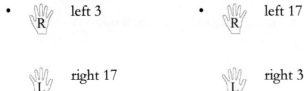

- left 3
- left 17

right 17

right 3

To understand correlations see:
- Organ flows: spleen, small intestines
- Energy locks: 3, 7

Nose

Nearly everyone has experienced nasal congestion and knows how unpleasant it is! Children, however, often don't complain because they don't know how it feels to have a free nose for they are used to their adenoids. If the nasal cavity is not sufficiently free it can lead to pain like headaches. Lack of moisture causes a dry mucous membrane. Drinking a lot of water and saline rinses are very helpful.

To harmonize:
- Hold ring fingers

- 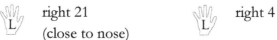 left 4

- left 21 (close to nose)

right 21 (close to nose)

right 4

To understand correlations see:
- Organ flows: stomach, bladder, colon, lungs
- Energy locks: 4, 9

Oedema - Edema

An oedema is a swelling due to accumulation of liquids in the tissue. There are many explanations for this condition and it should be evaluated by a physician. Practicing Jin Shin Jyutsu will aid in supporting free flow. Two very important organs are the kidneys and the bladder. Both belong to the element water.

Moving in fresh air strengthens the circulation and via muscle movement tissue liquids are mobilized. This again stabilizes the heart. Elevation of swollen feet and legs helps the blood flow back to the heart. Orthopaedic or reinforced leggings are also a good supportive alternative.

To harmonize:
- Hold index fingers

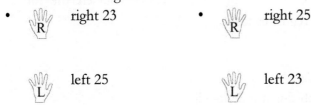

- right 23
- right 25

  left 25
  left 23

To understand correlations see:
- Organ flows: bladder, kidneys
- Energy lock: 23

Overweight

This topic is very common. Diets promise weight loss and when the promise is not fulfilled, followers are disappointed. Much has been written about the 'yo-yo effect'. This is the up and down, down and up experienced with many diets. The mechanism behind this is that the body learns to tolerate less food. And since the body does not forget anything, it immediately stores deposits for bad times. By losing weight, muscle tissue breaks down and is rebuilt as fat tissue immediately when not exercising. This demonstrates how dangerous slimming diets can be, because the heart is also a muscle.

Appropriate exercise in fresh air is therefore essential for any kind of dietetic experiments in order to train and strengthen the heart muscle. Remember to practice Jin Shin Jyutsu. The more harmonizing energy flows within yourself the more your weight regulates itself.

To harmonize:
- Hold each finger individually

-

To understand correlations see:
- Organ flows: stomach, kidneys, gall bladder
- Energy locks: 21, 23

Pain

Tolerance to pain is very different for each individual and gives no reliable conclusion of an illness. Scientific research attempts to discover the phenomenon of pain. There is an association set up for pain therapies and specifically established pain clinics.

Also Jin Shin Jyutsu offers measures for pain relief. First of all the main central flow and the self embracement (big hug) gives the initial boost. In addition see at the specified keywords.

To harmonize:
- Hold hands cross wise on the pain (L on top of R)
- Hold fingertips of both hands right and left of the vertex (= crown)
- 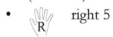 right 5

  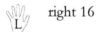 right 16

- 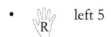 left 5

   left 16

To understand correlations see:
- Organ flow: stomach
- Energy lock: 5, 14, 16

Posture

Posture is an expression of the person's inner attitude. What should good posture look like? Keep your feet flat on the floor with your weight equally distributed on both feet. Maintain an erect position and be conscious of your breast bone and stick out your chest. This initiates a tension at the lumbar vertebra and your abdomen automatically gets stretched. Drop your shoulders.

Notice how relaxed you feel and enjoy your straight posture.

Hint: Remember throughout the day to consider your posture – while standing, sitting or walking. Even when lying down you can lift your breast bone by pushing the shoulders down.

To harmonize:
* Hold each finger individually
* 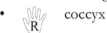 coccyx

 each vertebra of neck

To understand correlations see:
* Main central flow
* Energy locks: 2, 13

Pregnancy

We know that the course of pregnancy is the basis for new human life, both on the physical and psychological level. Medical science has established the precise developmental stages of nascent human beings. That means we can help the embryo in its specific development with appropriate Jin Shin Jyutsu treatments.

To harmonize:
- Hold each finger individually
- Hold both 13
- Hold both 26

To understand correlations see:
- Organ flows: liver, lung, spleen
- Energy locks: 4, 9

Prostate

The prostate has the tendency to enlarge with age and puts strain on the urethra. Nowadays it happens frequently even in younger men, for which there are various reasons. But one reason we know for sure is the prostate does not like the moist heat in too tight pants. The old knights may already have known this as we can conclude from the shape of their clothes. A lot of drinking, cold showers and chewing pumpkin seeds are the best method besides Jin Shin Jyutsu as a prophylaxis to prevent enlargement of the prostate.

To harmonize:
- Hold both 8
- Main central flow

To understand correlations see:
- Organ flows: kidneys, bladder
- Energy lock: 8

Rage

This emotion is interrelated with the liver and gall-bladder.

It can be a physical condition which expresses itself through rage but it can also be a characteristic emotion that, in the long run, burdens the liver and the gall-bladder. Rage can be a source for physical discomfort. In any case, this emotion needs harmonizing because the affected person will suffer from his long-term enduring rage and so will the people around him.

To harmonize:
- Hold middle fingers
- Hold both 14 – also cross wise

To understand correlations see:
- Organ flows: liver, gall bladder, spleen
- Energy lock: 14

Relaxation -> see: Insomnia - Relaxation

Rheumatism

The term rheumatism is an outdated term for dragging and coursing pain, and is blamed for a variety of discomforts: Pain in tendons, muscles, joints, bursa and the musculoskeletal system. The term arthritis is defined and related to inflammatory processes in the joints. To activate a perfect energy flow we need a special nutrition besides drinking plenty of water and of course Jin Shin Jyutsu.

To harmonize:
- Hold each finger individually

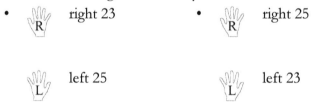

-     right 23   •   right 25

-     left 25   left 23

To understand correlations see:
- Organ flows: kidneys, bladder, liver, gall bladder
- Energy lock: 23

Sacrum

In most cases when we suffer from low-back pain we concentrate on this area instead of checking the entire spine. The spine is shaped like an 'S' in order to balance movement, posture and weight. But lower back pain primarily includes tension in the shoulder girdle, for which the spine compensates. Therefore pay attention to your posture and relax your back while practicing Jin Shin Jyutsu.

To harmonize:
* Hold each finger individually

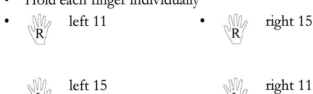

left 11	right 15
left 15	right 11

* on pain affected area

above

To understand correlations see:
* Organ flows: bladder, kidneys, gall bladder
* Energy lock: 2

Sadness

A person with grief and sadness usually lets his shoulders and head hang low. Thus the lungs can no longer receive the abundance of fresh air because the view is pointed to the ground. There is nothing wrong with establishing an appropriate space for sadness in order to look at it with awareness and experience its extent in order to overcome it in due course. Then we can stand up again and are not absorbed by it any longer. Jin Shin Jyutsu helps handling the sadness.

To harmonize:
- Hold ring fingers
- Hold both 15
- Hold both 22

To understand correlations see:
- Organ flows: lung, large intestine
- Energy locks: 9, 13

Sciatica -> see: Lumbago

Shock

The reflex reaction to a shock is immediately taking a deep breath and not exhaling completely. With this accumulated air the shock remains stuck in us. Also attending a loved person that is going through lingering illness or is close to death can cause rigidity in us as we do not exhale properly and can result in a long-term shock condition. With our hands, we can solve these blockages and let love and light flow into the inner darkness allowing us to experience the process more easily.

To harmonize:
- Hold middle fingers
- Hold both 7

To understand correlations see:
- Organ flows: stomach, spleen
- Energy lock: 4
- Main central flow

Shoulders

We carry our burdens, our worries and our responsibilities on our shoulders. In order to better balance the weight we pull up our shoulders. This places the neck in an awkward wrong position. Eventually the shoulders ache, which is no wonder on account of their inappropriate position. It is certainly clear that this long process can definitively not be cured or corrected with one or two injections. Practice dropping your shoulders. Free yourself of all the unnecessary baggage. Mary Burmeister says: *"Be simply the dropping of your shoulders."*

To harmonize:
- Hold each finger individually

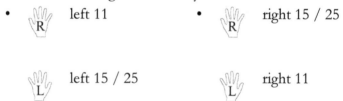

-   left 11   •   right 15 / 25

  left 15 / 25   right 11

To understand correlations see:
- Organ flows: large intestine, small intestine
- Energy locks: 11, 12

Skin

The skin is our biggest organ with a variety of tasks, for example thermal regulation, excretion, absorption and protection including a reflection of our inner emotional life. It is a sensorial organ that perceives and reacts very sensitively towards our environment. Certain skin areas indicate possible disharmony in the organ system. A change in appearance can also reflect changes in the body's system.

The skin actually is a life-sustaining respiratory organ. Since the skin constantly renews itself, we have the opportunity to enhance our well being by following a balanced diet and including outdoor activities.

Hint: Take warm and cold showers and massage your skin with a brush.

To harmonize:
- Hold each finger individually
- Hold both 8

To understand correlations see:
- Organ flows: stomach, spleen, lung, colon
- Energy lock: 8

Slipped Disc

Slipped discs are usually caused by the bilateral muscle cords unequally tugging at the spine. Even a small but permanent pressure, like a swollen liver, can cause an imbalance as mentioned above. Psychological pressure can also lead to severe discomfort.

Basically our posture is the expression of our inner attitude. The following exercises are recommended to do repeatedly:

- Straighten your breast bone and stretch the head softly and smoothly upwards.
- Feel inside, the flow of the central vitality descending in front and ascending in back.
- Try to breathe into the painful spot.

At the beginning you might have difficulties with this straight posture for the muscles are not yet used to support the spine.

Hint: Take a convenient posture like sitting, standing or lying down. Place the right hand on the aching area and the left hand crosswise on top, either with the palm or with the back of the hand.

Hint: Help yourself with a pillow under the lower back while sitting and while lying with a rolled up towel.

To harmonize:
- Hold all fingers individually

- left 11
- right 15

left 15

right 11

To understand correlations see:
- Organ flows: bladder, liver, gall bladder
- Energy lock: 2
- Finger-Toe-Flow (see: Finger)

Snoring

Snoring is noisy breathing caused by the fluttering movements of the relaxed soft palate / velum or through a dropped tongue. But this is of no interest to the person next to a snorer who becomes more and more alert and angry. Put your hands carefully on the snorer in a way that is most comfortable for you.

To harmonize:
- Hold middle finger either left or right

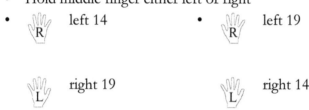

-     left 14
-     left 19

    right 19   right 14

To understand correlations see:
- Organ flows: stomach, spleen
- Energy lock: 14

Spasms

Spasms are involuntarily muscle convulsions of different origins and effects, e.g. lack of oxygen, mineral imbalance, too much acidity, muscle strain and energy blockages caused by scars.

Almost always the quality of one's blood or an imbalanced energy flow has an influence on spasms.

To harmonize:
• Hold both 23

Tummy cramps:

• R	left 11	• R	right 25
L	left 25	L	right 11

Cramps in the calf:

• R	right 8	• R	left 16
L	right 16	L	left 8

To understand correlations see:
• Organ flows: kidneys, bladder, spleen, gall bladder
• Energy lock: 8

Stomach Ache

Stomach ache, gas and spasms are experienced by many people who have a weak gastro-intestinal tract. Too much raw and cold food, cold beverages and too much dairy, burden the gastro-intestinal tract, because harmful waste remains in the system. A specified, adjusted food change will be beneficial. While practicing Jin Shin Jyutsu, motion and noises in the intestines are a welcome indication for an improvement.

To harmonize:
- Hold little finger
- Both hands crosswise placed on the abdomen (L on top of R)

- left 11
- right 25

left 25

right 11

To understand correlations see:
- Organ flows: stomach, spleen, liver
- Energy lock: 14
- See also: Spasms

Stress

The word 'stress' is on everyone's lips; even school children suffer from it. A healthy stress unleashes forces and inspires creativity. Negative experienced stress blasts the nerves and causes illness. Therefore the word 'stress' should not be used in our daily speech in order to avoid creating a negative atmosphere.

By practicing regularly Jin Shin Jyutsu stress is reduced and we are harmonized.

To harmonize:
*   Hold each finger individually
*   Main central flow

To understand correlations see:
*   Organ flows: stomach, spleen, small intestine
*   Energy locks: 14, 17, 23

Sweating -> see: Feeling Cold

Teeth – Gums – Dental Pain

Our teeth cause us pain when they come– and again when they leave. In between, they help us bite and chew food. When the effort of 'biting through' is too great, the teeth react audibly with grinding.

Through the years they suffer in silence through grinding while passing on their discomfort to the body's internal organs. Teeth are hard on their exterior but internally they are quite sensitive. When experiencing tooth aches and bleeding gums, medical care is necessary and additional Jin Shin Jyutsu practices are helpful.

To harmonize:

- Hold thumbs
- Hold index fingers

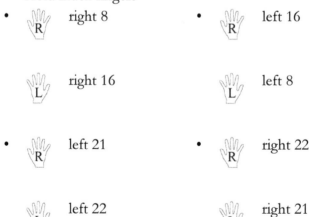

-    R   right 8
-    R   left 16

   L   right 16   L   left 8

-    R   left 21
-    R   right 22

   L   left 22   L   right 21

To understand correlations see:
- Organ flows: stomach, kidneys, large intestines
- Energy locks: 8, 21

Third Eye

Our third eye is located between the eye brows. Sensible and experienced people have strong perceptions. This is an important cross point of many different energy flows which we can harmonize by simply holding it.

To harmonize:
- First step of central flow

To understand correlations see:
- Organ flow: small intestines
- Energy lock: 20

Thoughts

There is a saying: 'Thoughts are free'. But in general we only 'think about' what has already been thought for us e.g. what to eat, drink, smoke, dress or believe in. Today free thoughts have become an illusion, for it is difficult to follow one's own path with one's own thoughts.

When Jin Shin Jyutsu is practiced daily, the development of our own thoughts and our independence is promoted.

To harmonize:
*   Self embracement (big hug) and the 36 conscious breaths
*   Main central flow

To understand correlations see:
*   Organ flows: stomach, heart
*   Energy locks: 21, 20

Throat -> see: Neck - Throat

Thyroid - Parathyroid

The thyroid holds a very important place in the regulation of all glands, from the pituitary gland to the periphery. It determines the basal energy production, which is necessary in maintaining the function of the organs and the metabolism. The parathyroid gland is involved in this complicated regulation system. One of its main tasks is the control of calcium and magnesium supply, especially important in menopause.

To harmonize:
- Hold thumbs
- right high 22
  behind the collar bone

   right arm pit

To understand correlations see:
- Organ flow: stomach
- Energy lock: 22

Tonsils – Inflammation

Mothers can tell a thing or two about swollen tonsils and sudden fever. Each time it is a question whether to consult or not to consult a physician because it might be more serious than the last time. First try clarifying the situation with Jin Shin Jyutsu and afterwards consult a physician if necessary.

To harmonize:
- Hold both 4
- 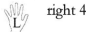 left 4
- left 21

 right 21

 right 4

To understand correlations see:
- Organ flows: lung, stomach
- Energy locks: 4, 21

Tummy Ache -> see: Stomach Ache

Varicose Veins

Varicose veins are prominent, visible vessels prevailing in women and also in men more than 50 years old. They are related to a slow back flow of the blood. Causes are many, for instance hereditary vessel membrane weakness, venous valve insufficiency, pregnancy or a hip imbalance. Especially at risk are those who are on their feet for extended periods, e.g. supermarket cashiers and waiters. Truck and bus drivers also have a high incidence of varicose vein problems.

Varicose veins are not a question of beauty standards, they should be watched carefully. Recommendations are alternating hot and cold foot baths, compresses and / or supportive orthopaedic leggings. We recommend elevated legs and practicing Jin Shin Jyutsu to enhance the metabolic system.

To harmonize:
- Place little finger on opposite big toe
- left 3
- right 15

 left 15

 right 3

- left 15

- right 2

left 2

right 15

To understand correlations see:
- Organ flows: spleen, kidneys
- Energy locks: 15, 23

Vitality

Vitality, nowadays, is the epitome of life and experience.

The vitality of our parents made us come into this world. We are a part of creation, a part of interaction between man and woman and of the process of growing and being. This deep memory leaves us longing for love in our lives. We search for love in which we are allowed to merge with the creation. These correlations are experienced with Jin Shin Jyutsu in its daily practice.

The central flow provides us with the needed energy at any moment. According to our possibilities, we can receive and develop this energy. The spleen energy nourishes us with the earth forces; the stomach frees our head from fixed patterns and the kidney energy comes with the vital contingent that we maintain when practicing Jin Shin Jyutsu.

To harmonize:
- Main central flow
- Hold each finger individually
- Self embracement (big hug) and the 36 conscious breaths

To understand correlations see:
- Organ flows: spleen, stomach, kidneys
- Energy locks: 19, 26

Weight

What is the ideal weight? Who hasn't experienced this ongoing battle, which can lead to a guilty conscience or even worse, to depression.

First we go into the kitchen to binge and this makes us feel better. Afterwards however, frustration sets in and in order to cheer us up, we go back to the kitchen and therefore we establish a continuous vicious circle. Jin Shin Jyutsu doesn't promise that you will reach your desired weight right away, but it will contribute decisively in stabilizing and balancing your inner condition. Slowly those eating attacks will stop and with confidence you will gain your desired weight.

To harmonize:

- Hold all fingers individually

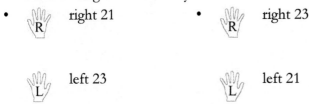

- right 21
- right 23
- left 23
- left 21

To understand correlations see:

- Organ flow: stomach
- Energy locks: 9, 14, 21, 22

Worries

Worry about the future, worry about the past, worry about the present, this is what concerns us daily. Worry is a kind of fear and accompanies or preoccupies us throughout our entire life. The constant concern burdens the earth element which is connected to the energy of stomach and spleen functions and destroys our sense of basic trust on the spiritual level.

Children sucking their thumb, intuitively harmonize their energy level, although it may not be beneficial in the long run neither for the thumb nor the growing teeth.

To harmonize:
- Hold thumbs

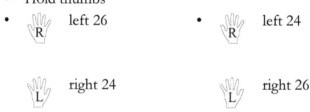

-   left 26
-   left 24

  right 24
  right 26

To understand correlations see:
- Organ flows: stomach, spleen
- Energy lock: 1

The 26 Energy Locks and Their Meaning

Pythagoras knew that: *"each number is a mystical creature with its distinctive vibration"*. That means numbers represent actions, fundamental principles of creation, which unfold through each individual number.

Each energy lock has an assigned number. Normally the series of numbers start at zero, called in the Japanese book of wisdom a 'cosmic egg'. It surrounds the human being and provides him with everything needed via the main central flow (see p. 20).

By practicing Jin Shin Jyutsu, the numbers slowly start to become familiar and we learn to experience them as energy locks. They make us more or less gently aware of those energy locks that should be 'oiled and opened'. They show us which body parts desire to be touched by our hands to come into harmony.

Learn about the Jin Shin Jyutsu numbers and become friends with them because they will open new spaces in your consciousness. Feel the wisdom when reading a short description of a number and get into contact with yourself and your inner wisdom. To one or the other number you will develop a stronger connection depending on your personal concern or anticipation.

In the following description, the significance of each individual numbers is explained. As already mentioned, an energy lock can either be open or locked without us noticing it as such.

The mentioned distinguishing characteristics associated with the individual numbers, can be the result of a blocked energy lock. It is essential to unblock the energy locks for energy to flow again. To do so, follow the listed practices. If you do not have specific symptoms, you can maintain each energy lock individually and thus remain in motion.

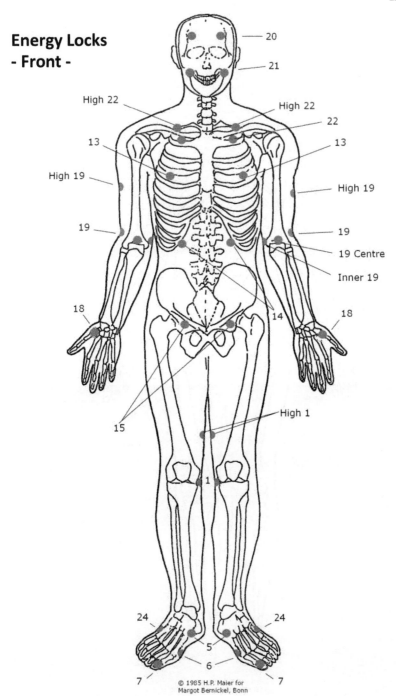

Energy Locks
- Front -

20
21
High 22
High 22
22
13
13
High 19
High 19
19
19
19 Centre
Inner 19
18
18
14
15
High 1
1
24
24
5
6
7
7

© 1985 H.P. Maier for
Margot Bernickel, Bonn

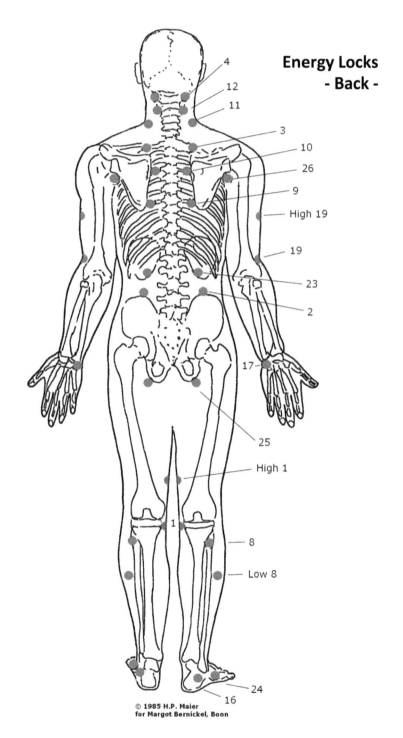

Energy Locks
- Back -

© 1985 H.P. Maier
for Margot Bernickel, Bonn

The 1 - One

The 1 is located on the inner knee and has the meaning: prime mover.

It is the unity of life and death of which a thought, an intention, an urge develops, like the knee which initiates our moves. The 1 helps exhale and releases blockages in the upper part of the body such as indigestion, bloating and constipation in the abdomen and head. When we breathe with awareness, locked in things are released and we then are able to receive the new.

The 1 embodies the solar principle. It is attributed to the male yang and helps our entire being including our health.

Support / Assistance:
- New start and to make progress – to go on -
- To free head and abdomen
- Self-awareness, worries
- Exhaling, swallowing, and hiccups
- Digestion

Practice:
- Hold thumbs
- Hold both 1
- 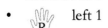 left 1   • 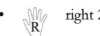 right 2

   left 2   right 1

The High 1 – One

The high 1 is about one hand above the 1 and is an important crossroad of multiple organ flows, easy to find because it is usually sensitive to the touch. The tension quickly dissolves through touch and will be very beneficial for you.

Support / Assistance:
- Cough
- Exhaling
- Swallowing
- Indigestion, nausea, stomach discomfort
- Sweets craving
- Weight

Practice:
- Hold both high 1 crosswise

The 2 - Two

The 2 is located at the upper hips and has the meaning: wisdom, life and vitality for all creatures.

The 2 protects the space in which new life is 'created'. Also described through the saying: 'look with the eyes of the Creator'. The 2 represents the feminine, the yin principle and the moon. The moon receives the light from the sun and reflects it. Receiving refers to both breathing in and to the ascending energy. This way the 2 helps with the ascending energy to free blockages or jams especially below the waist, like the legs, hips and back. It will help the spine to straighten; expecting mothers know this intuitively by placing their hands on the 2. 'As above, so below' is an important principle, even with Jin Shin Jyutsu. When the energy can ascend at the back it can also descend at the front. Through a released 2 respiration and digestion become flawless.

Support / Assistance:
- Inhaling, receiving
- Accepting, to accept oneself
- Spine, body structure, intervertebral disc, back, bones, osteoporosis
- Tension in legs
- Posture

Practice:
- Hold ring fingers
- Hold both 2

-  left 3   • right 2

  left 2   right 3

The 3 - Three

The 3 is located at the top of the back between shoulder blades and spine and has the meaning: door, understanding, defence.

The 3 is responsible for both inhalation and exhalation. As a swinging door it allows our breath to come and go and releases all the tensions, scepticism and old breath to receive new, clean energy.

The 3 will be referred to as our respiratory specialist because it protects the upper points of our lungs, which only a few people are aware of, for example singers and meditating people. An inappropriate posture and breathing burden the 3 and cause a jammed door. The air cannot flow properly in and out to cleanse and renew us. Only with a strong and healthy breathing our immune system can develop effectively. Therefore the 3 is also designated as our natural antibiotic. Inhaling and exhaling represent taking and giving on all levels. Our breath is the ultimate healer and promotes our balance mentally and physically.

Support / Assistance:
- Inhaling and exhaling
- Bronchus, lungs, mucus
- Immune system, lymph, nerves
- Sore throat
- Shoulder, neck, arms and all fingers
- Colds, flu, fever
- Congestion in the groin and feet

Practice:
- Hold middle fingers
- Hold both 3
-  left 3

- right 15

  left 15

  right 3

- right 3

- thumb on each fingernail

  thumb on each fingernail

  left 3

The 4 - Four

The 4 is located at the base of the skull in the dimples right and left of the neck and has the meaning: window.

At the 4 many nerves and vessels come out of the head and go back inside again. These energy locks are a bridge between the visible and invisible, between formlessness and form, between mind and body.

They check 144,000 special body functions and provide a regulation. They take care of the transition between wakefulness and sleep, coming and going. The 4 brings the awareness into the physicality and also withdraws it.

Support / Assistance:
- Eyes
- View (clear sight, insight, to look through)
- Nose and sinuses
- Neck tension
- Deep fatigue, insomnia, pregnancy
- Headaches, migraines, dizziness
- Shock
- Tonsillitis

Practice:
- Hold ring fingers
- Hold both 4

- left 4
- left 21

 right 21

 right 4

The 5 - Five

The 5 is located inside the ankle joint, between ankle and heel and has the meaning: renewal, solving fear.

It helps us to release the old and makes room to receive the new.

The 5 is the symbolic number for man who is the connection between the elements and spirit.

We have 5 fingers on each hand and 5 toes on each foot and 5 senses in our consciousness. The 5 asks us to perceive the senses but not to be dominated by them. So it is possible to gradually let go of fear that ties us to the past and prevents the new.

Releasing fear gives us the power to live freely.

Support / Assistance:
- Fear
- Pain
- Lack of energy
- Clear chest
- Clear shoulders
- Clear hearing, ears
- Dropping the old and accepting the new
- Digestion
- Regeneration and change of the consciousness

Practice:
- Hold index fingers

-   R   right 15   •   R   left 3

      L   right 3   L   left 15

-   R   right 15   •   R   left 5

      L   right 5   L   left 15

-   R   right 5   •   R   left 16

      L   right 16   L   left 5

The 6 - Six

The 6 is located in our longitudinal foot arch and has the meaning: balance, discrimination.

As a bridge is supported through an arch, so is our body through our foot arch and erected via the spine. The erect position of our spine with its S-shape is very important for our balance-organ in the ear. Only in balance we find our own level and recognize that of others. This way the ability of distinction and judgment without rating is gradually developed which is essential for the internal balance. This way contrasting experiences are interconnected.

Support / Assistance:
- Spine, bone structure, osteoporosis
- Back, hip
- Shoulders, arms, hands
- Lungs
- Digestion
- Fungus
- Grounding
- Harmony, balance, dizziness, understanding

Practice:
- Hold middle fingers

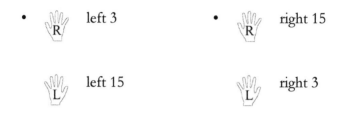

- 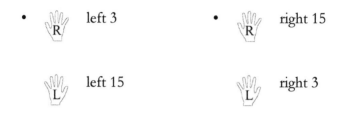 left 3
- 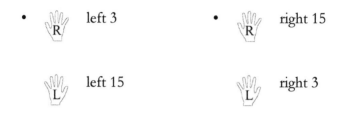 right 15

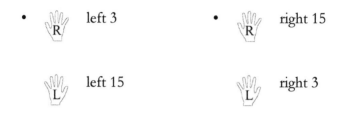 left 15

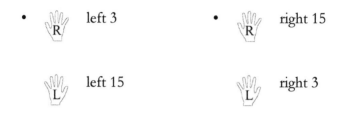 right 3

- Hold 6 and 24 comfortably with both hands on the same foot

The 7 - Seven

The 7 is located at the bottom of the big toe and has the meaning: victory, perfect vitality.

When the descending energy finally comes to the toe, victory and vitality are in perfect flow from head to toe. Many people know from foot-reflexology that the big toe relieves and clears the head and allows a spiritual development. Please watch the shoe-fashion!

The 7 is of great significance because we know 7 laws of life, 7 days, 7 basic elements, 7 crystal systems and many more.

The 7 transforms the descending energy during a short pause into the ascending energy.

Support / Assistance:
- Head clearing, nausea, dizziness
- Respiratory problems, asthma, hay fever, allergy
- State of shock
- Chest pressure
- Digestion
- Grounding

Practice:
- Hold ring fingers
- Hold both 7

-    right 15

      left 2

-    right 7

      right 8

-    right 2

      left 15

-    left 8

      left 7

The 8 - Eight

The 8 is located lateral at the back of the knee and has the meaning: rhythm, strength, peace.

It is the highest 'female' number. The 8 combines, in itself, heaven and earth forces which it brings to mankind. What was up is down the next moment and what is inside is now outside. In its curves of two circles with no beginning and no ending lies the potential of vitality. Especially to draw the lying 8 into the air with folded hands brings rhythm to the being and gives inner peace. This is a very important practice for dyslexia, as it also links both brain halves with each other.

The 8 is located on the leg where we tighten our muscles in the western world to stand at attention. In the eastern tradition, people learn to relax their muscles in the 8 to be anchored and grounded to withstand storms more easily (e.g. in Tai Chi).

The 8 takes care of the skin and brings the inside to the outside.

Support / Assistance:
- Muscle tension, calf cramps, stiffness
- Skin problems, acne, burns, radiation damage
- Intake and excretion (diarrhoea and constipation)
- Reproduction
- Pelvic girdle, prostate

Practice:
- Hold index fingers
- Hold both 8

- 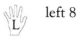 right 25

  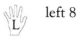 left 25

- 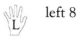 left little toe

  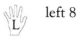 left 8

- right 8

   right little toe

When experiencing diarrhoea:
- right 8

   left 2

When experiencing constipation:
- right 2

   left 8

The 9 - Nine

The 9 is located between spine and shoulder blade tip and has the meaning: the end of a cycle and the beginning of a new.

That means 'the end of life of the caterpillar is a new beginning for the butterfly'. It also symbolizes that in each end there is already the germ of something new and in each beginning there already is the end ingrained.

The 9 contains the ageless wisdom: we are at the same time the past, the present and even the future. It helps to understand ourselves and our own state of being.

The 9 helps us to draw a final line under the past and to start over again. On the physical level the 9 takes care of the extremities, including arms and legs and supports the ascending energy.

It is difficult to touch the 9 with our own hands, as we often have difficulties to enter new shores in particular life situations. With our own eyes we cannot see the 9 without an auxiliary medium (mirror, person) as we cannot discover our shadow-sides alone (therapy, self experience).

Support / Assistance:
- Congestion in the chest
- Back, hips, legs, feet
- Respiratory, asthma, frontal sinuses, sinuses of the nose, hay fever, allergy
- Colon, excretion
- Head, blood pressure
- Change of circumstances, pregnancy
- Growth

Practice:

- Hold thumbs
- Hold both elbows
- Hold both upper arms on the 9 altitude
- left elbow
- left 14
  (costal arch)

 right 14
(costal arch)

 right elbow

The 10 - Ten

The 10 is located between the spine and the middle of the shoulder blade and the spine and has the meaning: outpouring of boundless vitality, reservoir of abundance.

The 10 is located at the height of the heart which is the seismograph of all matters in our life. When we are in love – and see things through rose coloured glasses, we feel a boundless vitality and love as if we could lift the world off its hinges. In the same way, our vitality is repressed when our heart is burdened. The 10 consists of the 1 and the 0. Their sum is 1, which demonstrates the close relation between these two numbers. The abundance of potential in the 0 is also included in the 10. In the free-flowing 10 vibrates male and female energy in equal shares and brings balance and harmony. The 10 is the higher frequency of the 1 with the experiences of the 1. All the heart matters we experience during our life remain stored in our billions of cells. Our 10 fingers, 10 toes and the 10 Commandments remind us of the importance of this number.

Support / Assistance:
- Matters of the heart, feelings
- Heart, view, eyes, vision, open the voice
- Dizziness
- Blood pressure, kidneys
- Tension in chest
- Breath, circulation
- Knee, hips, neck, shoulders
- Mind, learning (dyslexia)

Practice:
- Hold index fingers
- Hold both upper arms on the 10 altitude
- left upper arm   • left thigh

       right thigh   right upper arm

The 11 - Eleven

The 11 is located between the angle of the neck and the shoulder and has the meaning: justice, unloading excess baggage.

Who does not drag old loads around which we try to balance with a yoke on our shoulders, like experienced injustice, unkindness or maybe sadness? Responsibility is also connected to a load, often demonstrated by shoulder decorations (e.g. uniforms with shoulder clasps, cords, etc.).

All burden and excess baggage manifested in the 11 may also be unloaded, which is one of our most important tasks in life. The 11 is the master key for all energy locks and for all flows. Almost all flows stream through the 11, they take care of proper breathing, digestion, intake, excretion and circulation, provided it is free of ballast.

Support / Assistance:
- Head, neck, shoulders, arms, hands, fingers
- Thoracic region
- Hip region, legs, lumbago, sciatica, legs
- Blood, blood vessels
- Digestive organs, pancreas
- Guilt, fear, efforts
- Decision making power

Practice:
- Hold index fingers

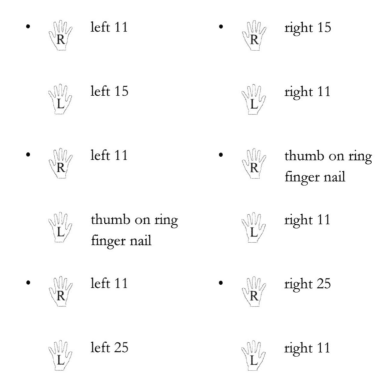

- left 11

  left 15

- left 11

  thumb on ring finger nail

- left 11

  left 25

- right 15

  right 11

- thumb on ring finger nail

  right 11

- right 25

  right 11

The 12 - Twelve

The 12 is located in the neck right and left of the spine at the fourth neck vertebrae and means: 'Thy will be done', the realignment with the universal will – in accordance with the law of nature.

Japanese bow their head and in doing this, the other person is honoured. This gesture of greeting is interpreted as 'I greet the Creator living in you'.

The opening of a conversation with bowing one's head facilitates coming into contact with the other partner and creates attention to listening. It is not surprising that the 12 helps to balance emotions, to clear the head for great ideas and the awareness of the universal existence. The 12 represents vitality; it makes the force of circumstances simple, like a surfer uses natural forces of wind and water to glide easily.

Support / Assistance:
- Back of the neck, neck, shoulder, arm, finger
- Opens waistline
- Sciatica, lumbago
- Clears head
- Blocked emotions
- Entanglement in fixed life style
- Whiplash trauma

Practice:
- Hold middle fingers
- Hold both 12

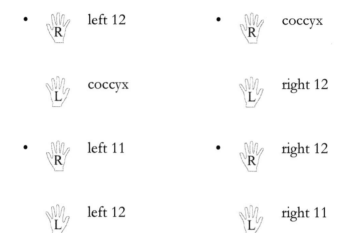

- left 12
  coccyx

- left 11
  left 12

- coccyx
  right 12

- right 12
  right 11

The 13 – Thirteen

The 13 is located to the left and right of the sternum centre and means: Open your heart also to people thinking differently, fertility and fountain of youth.

The 13 is at the height of the heart and takes care of all heart matters. There our feelings of guilt are stuck, there we ask for forgiveness and there we experience a feeling of being new born, similar to a heart immersed in joy.

In Tarot the 13 symbolizes death which means change including making space for the new.

Something new is born when we dissolve jammed feelings as in anger, hatred and guilt. Love now flows once again from the heart. Therefore the 13 reenergizes power on each level and brings awareness of spirit and spirituality. It makes us grow in each aspect and harmonizes the environment we are living in. The 13 is by no means an occupied negative number but on the contrary reflects our divine soul.

Mary Burmeister says: *"Be the fountain and not the reservoir."*

Support / Assistance:
- Chest level, shoulder, neck
- Respiratory, immune system, cancer
- Thyroid glands, metabolism
- Reproductive functions, women issues
- Regenerative power, love-life
- All mucous membranes, abdomen
- Mental and emotional tensions
- Posture
- Spirituality

Practice:
- Hold index finger
- Hold middle finger
- Hold little finger
- Hold both upper arms
- 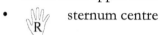 sternum centre

 pubic bone

The 14 - Fourteen

The 14 is located in the middle of the body right and left at the rib cage and means: balance, sustenance.

In the waist area the digestive tract produces the liquids; the 14 oversees the processing of food we consume as a material and immaterial substance. The human being does not live from bread alone but also depends on smelling, viewing, reading, feeling, tasting, hearing and thinking. The 14 is the expression of the human being, with his willpower, who embodies the combination 'as above so below', heaven and earth. In this area the spirit transforms into materialization.

A blocked 14 can cause reverse energy leading to serious consequences from snoring to unconsciousness. Therefore it is advisable to avoid heavy food especially at night.

The 14 guards the much discussed solar plexus, where the sun organ, the spleen, absorbs all radiation to direct it to the other organs and nerves. Here we do not only absorb the good sunrays but also those not always beneficial to us. That's why we defend the 14 intuitively with our hands.

Support / Assistance:
- Harmony between top and bottom
- Snoring and nightmares, asthma
- Hiccups
- Stagnation in head
- Teeth grinding
- Hip, cold, swollen feet, cramps
- Heart complaints, guilt
- Stomach pain, abdominal discomfort, bloating

- Lump in the throat, rage
- Sweating, relieving stress
- Grounding

Practice:
- Hold ring fingers
- Hold both elbows
- Hold both 14 cross wise
- Hold both 12
- 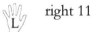 left 19

- 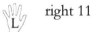 left high 1 (thigh)

   right high 1 (thigh)

   right 19

- left 11

- right 14

   left 14

   right 11

The 15 - Fifteen

The 15 is located in the groin and means: wash your heart with laughter.

The 15 is the joy and laughter itself. When the heart laughs with joy, 'when we see the world through rose coloured glasses', or simply put, when we are in love; then the groin would like to resonate with us, with our heart.

This close relationship between heart and groin also counts in other cases: namely when the heart is burdened and symptoms show up, the groin must be released in order to let all accumulations descend. This makes the heart free for the joy to come.

Here it becomes clear how close the links between the different levels are: The 13 area at heart level is the level of consciousness, the 15 area at groin level is the body level. The 14 area at waist level is the expression of the human's mind and his level of understanding. It is his connection between 13 and 15. Thus the physicality is the lowest form of spirituality and the spirituality the highest form of physicality. The laughter of the 15 cleanses and washes our being with all its thoughts, feelings and physical sensitivities.

The U.S. physician Dr. Norman Cousins, once seriously ill, practiced the healing of laughter in a self-experiment and wrote a book about his findings.

The 15 has the sum of the digits 1 and 5 = 6, which means balance. The 1 in the 15 contains the whole and represents divinity and the 5 the human being. In laughter these different levels are connected.

Support / Assistance:
- Tension in lower abdomen, legs, hips, knees, feet
- Heart rhythm, vascular system
- Sprains, fractures
- Surgeries
- Digestion, bloating
- Balance
- Back pain
- Gout
- Varicose veins

Practice:
- Hold little fingers
- Hold both 15
- 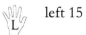 left 3

   left 15

- left 11

   left 15

- 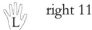 right 15

   right 3

- right 15

   right 11

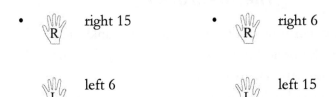

- right 15

- left 6

- right 6

- left 15

The 16 - Sixteen

The 16 is located at the foot between the outer ankle and heel and means: the basic foundation for our being, actions and transformation, a bridge to activity.

Life is change and only in the constant change our inner core can move outward, penetrating the entire being and become identical with it. The 16 helps us to gradually clean the accumulated layers and to build something new.

In foot reflexology the area around the 16 is known for its close relation to the ovaries, testes and reproduction. The 16 clarifies and renews the thinking and consequently one's actions.

Emotional and physical injuries and their scars can be changed by holding the 16 and the area of the scar. Altered thinking also creates a modified tissue and a change in character qualities. The 16 with its sum of digits of 1 and 6 = 7 (meaning victory) makes clear that we can be victorious if we face the change and break old patterns.

Support / Assistance:
- Clear thinking, logical understanding, frontal headaches, migraine
- Voice, speech, dyslexia
- Neck stiffness, general muscle tensions, calf cramps, stiffness
- Scars (one hand on the scar, the other on the 16)
- Reproduction
- Arthritis, phantom pain
- Bones

- Excretion
- Jaw pain (one hand on jaw, the other on the 16)

Practice:
- Hold thumbs
- right 16   • left little toe

   right little toe   left 16

Speciality: Pain-Stop
- right 5   • left 5

   right 16   left 16

  In both cases R on the 5!

Speciality: Muscle Tension
- right 8   • left 16

   right 16   left 8

The 17 – Seventeen

The 17 is located on the side of the wrist and means: relaxation of mind and nerves, intuition and reproductive energy.

The location of the 17 is not very spectacular – one initially thinks so. The 17 is the sum of the digits of 1 and 7 = 8, this wonderful magic number is associated with eternity as is the 17. The intuition of the 17 recalls our source of eternity, the eternally valid law. From there flows the unlimited renewed energy. The 17 is the number of the zodiac Aquarius, which dissolves boundaries.

Our mind and nerves can calm down when facing a higher order, which even acts supportive while one is unconscious. The touch of the 17 – also used in the Buddhist meditation posture - together with the 16 helps to clear thinking and gain access to universal intelligence.

Mary Burmeister said: *"Be simple and the answer will come."* That means the 17 gives us the spiritual aspect of our actions. Public speakers and elderly people very frequently hold their 17. It has a close connection to the heart, which on a physical level is our life-giver and also represents mind and heart of all matters.

Support / Assistance:
* Breathing, sleep disturbances
* Heart and sternum
* Nerves and vascular system, releasing stress
* Emergency
* Ankles

- Bloating
- Opening the mind, creativity

Practice:
- Hold ring fingers
- Hold little fingers
- Hold both 17

The 18 – Eighteen

The 18 is located in the metacarpus joint of the thumb and means: body awareness and functions that affect the human personality.

What does this mean? Let us remember that the thumb harmonizes concern and worries, representing the basic trust. With this it means; if I have basic trust I am in my centre. I stand upright and have a healthy body awareness that feeds all my 27 million body cells, bringing me into balance and giving me a good rhythm. The sum of 18 is 9 on a different level; it ends a cycle and provides a bridge to another dimension. It helps us sleep well or stay awake. It is also the answer to the question of who we are and what the essence of our individuality in this life is.

Support / Assistance:
- Problem solving of any kind
- Back of head, feet
- Clears abdomen from head to toe
- Sternum, ribs
- Stiffness of back
- Insomnia
- Circulating thoughts

Practice:
- Hold thumbs
- Hold both 18

- left 3

- right 25

 left 25

 right 3

The 19 - Nineteen

The 19 is located on the thumb side in the elbow and means: authority, leadership ability, and perfect balance.

17, 18 and 19 are located at the arm, which represents the principle of action. The 19 thereby takes over the leadership, 18 stands for the mind and 17 for the spirit. If our actions are motivated and carried out with a clear spirit and mind then we personally take leadership and bring ourselves into perfect balance.

The sum of 19 = 10, which gives us the abundance of life, the 10 reduced to 1 brings the unity. All this is in the 19, which helps us to develop our personal responsibility for our life.

The position of 19 is known to many people – also to non-tennis players – as a painful tennis elbow. The reasons for this can be found, for example in the straining of the arm or an energy congestion in the 10. The 19 is so important that there is an additional energy lock known as high 19, which helps the upper back (at levels 9 and 10).

Support / Assistance:
- Chest, lungs, hiccups
- Arm, hand
- Leg backside
- Back pain
- Harmonizes both body halves and their energy

Practice:
- Hold thumbs

- Hold both 19 respective high 19
- left high 19
- lift high 1

 right high 1   right high 19

The 20 - Twenty

The 20 is located on the forehead over the eyebrows and means: perpetual, eternity.

The 20 is very familiar to us, for example when we unwittingly touch our forehead in a way to better concentrate or focus.

Also the act of 'tapping one's head' is an expression of deep significance of the 20. It leads us to see clearly, common sense and even knowledge of everlasting, valid principles and connections.

The 20 is also the 2 with the meaning to see the importance with new eyes. The 20 is the bridge between the personal and universal consciousness.

The 20 is our brain specialist that also calms the brain, so that we can let the everlasting wisdom penetrate into our consciousness.

Support / Assistance:
- Eye pain, eyelid, ear ache, balance
- Clear mental activity, consciousness
- Memory, migraine
- Chest, heart
- Bladder

Practice:
- Hold little fingers
- Hold both 20
- Hold both 22

- left high 19

 right high 1

- left high 1

right high 19

The 21 – Twenty-One

The 21 is located on the cheek below the cheek bone, and means: deep security, escape from mental bondage.

The meaning of 21 is demonstrated unconsciously by school children who, while exhausted, hang over their plate with their hands at 21, thus releasing their school worries and burdens. Here the stomach flow starts digestion of material and spiritual food.

There is a saying: 'A full stomach doesn't like to study'.

This means mental relaxation releases energy for physical digestion and also physical digestion is preparing a clear mind to strengthen the capacity of thought. A clear head frees us from mental or physical bondage.

Support / Assistance:
- Mental strain, fixed ideas, circular thoughts
- Depression, mood swings
- Unloading ballast on all levels
- Rosy cheeks (often symbolizes blocked energy)
- Drowsiness and dizziness
- Weight regulation, eating habits
- Eye relaxation
- Self-confidence

Practice:
- Hold thumbs
- Hold both 21

- 🤚 R   left high 1

🤚 L   right high 1

- 🤚 R   left 21   • 🤚 R   left high 1

🤚 L   right high 1   🤚 L   right 21

- 🤚 R   left 21   • 🤚 R   left 4

🤚 L   right 4   🤚 L   right 21

The 22 - Twenty-Two

The 22 is located below the collarbone and means: completeness, adaptation, crown of energy distribution.

In the 22 everything is included. It is the fusion of all elements, colours and sounds. Here is the place where all the pathways of the 144,000 special body functions are reorganized and harmonized. The energy that descends through the 22 relieves the head pressure and thus prevents even a stroke. It is an important cross road for our respiratory system which is supported by an upright position in this area. Furthermore the 22 harmonizes parathyroid and thyroid glands, also called our adaption organ. It influences our entire basal metabolic rate: the adaption of our cardio vascular system to the circumstances, for example the weather or other modified situations like our psychological and emotional concerns.

At the 20 we recognize our burdens, at the 21 we can let them go and at the 22 we learn something new.

As we exhale consciously, we receive twice, 22 in the doubling of the 2, which stands for inhalation. What great importance the 22 has, one can see at the burial posture of the pharaohs: crossed arms and hands on the 22. The 22 is also called a 'master number'.

Support / Assistance:
- Emotional and mental tensions
- Adaption and mediation
- Satisfaction and happiness
- Head pressure, stroke prevention

- Calcium and magnesium budget
- Hormone budget
- Thyroid, parathyroid glands
- Cough, lungs

Practice:
- Hold index fingers
- Hold both 22 crosswise
- right 11

- right 22

- left 19

 left 22

 left 11

 left high 1

right high 1

right 19

The 23 - Twenty-Three

The 23 is located on the back at the height of the kidneys and adrenal glands and means: maintaining the proper circulation, guard of human destiny.

The location of the 23 at the kidneys is significant for the importance of this 'energy security lock'. According to the Asian doctrine, the kidneys are the location of our inherited vitality, so we should handle them with care. The kidneys tirelessly filter our blood; their work is to preserve our life's vitality. Blood is the essence of our entire being. Today there are methods by which one drop of blood can provide information of various processes and circumstances in our body. When the body is poisoned we have poisonous thoughts. If the 23 is able to work in harmony, the kidneys can filter the blood appropriately. Thinking is then processed with more awareness and clarity.

The adrenal glands are adjacent to the kidneys. They are activated by a diversity of intense feelings. Under these conditions the adrenal glands secrete directly into the blood stream (e.g. escape behaviour). This makes clear that the 23 is the guard of our destiny. A free 23 enables us to perceive fear, face it and transform it into courage. Thus we practice tolerance and look at things from another point of view. The 23 is the key point of the water element and represents the flow of life.

Support / Assistance:
- All blood issues, gout, rheumatism, arthritis
- Consistency of blood, like diabetes, cholesterol, etc.

- Blood poison (drugs)
- Blood pressure, circulation
- Addictive behaviour, egoism
- Nervous tension, hyperactivity, stress reduction
- Unclear thinking
- Escape behaviour, eating habits
- Accumulation (tumours), oedema
- Obesity
- Hair, nails

Practice:
- Hold index fingers
- Hold little fingers
- Hold both 23
- right 23
- right 25

left 25

left 23

- right 21
- right 23

left 23

left 21

The 24 - Twenty-Four

The 24 is located on the foot in the hollow between the base of the three outer toes and the foot edge and means: understanding, peacemaker, harmonizing chaos.

At the Buddhist meditation posture the 24 (sum = 6, with the meaning 'balance') is placed on the opposite groin (15, sum = 6) and the back of the hand is placed in the arch of the foot (6). This induces harmony and balance on all levels. In this peaceful balance (if one is experienced!) the immensity of being reveals itself; chaos, jealousy, revenge and stubbornness have no place any longer.

Mary Burmeister said: *"The 24 helps us to grow and to become what we already are."*

Support / Assistance:
* Harmonizing chaos, hyperactivity
* Understanding and self-understanding
* Exhaustion and balance
* Jealousy, revenge, stubbornness

Practice:
* Hold little fingers
* Hold both 26 (embracing)

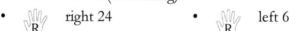

*   right 24   •   left 6

    right 6   left 24

• 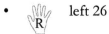 left 26

• left 24

 right 24

 right 26

The 25 - Twenty-Five

The 25 is located on the buttocks and means: regenerating quietly.

In many respiratory therapies the buttocks have a great importance. They serve the notion of forming additionally long roots towards the ground to get renewed by the earth forces. This renewal takes place at rest but equally while awake, and nourishes body, mind and spirit. According to a proverb: 'In calmness rests the power' or 'in peace lies the strength'.

Many people like to sit on their hands to warm them. But even without reason give it a try and get connected also mentally with the 25. You will notice the comforting feeling of having arrived home in yourself.

The 25 (sum = 7, means victory). Victories stimulate us positively, make us happy and set new energies free.

Support / Assistance:
- Inattention
- Circulation, blood pressure
- Sports, movement
- Chaotic spirit, overly excited
- Bundling of energy
- Problems become tasks

Practice:
- Hold middle fingers
- Hold both 25

- 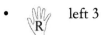 left 3

- 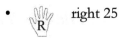 right 25

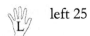 left 25

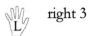 right 3

The 26 - Twenty-Six

The 26 is located at the outer edge of the shoulder blades and means: the director, complete, all that was, is and will be.

We touch the 26 (or as far as we can reach) in our daily self embracement with the 36 conscious breaths (see p. 19). This exercise brings us total harmony and vital life force for all mental and physical functions. Thus we become conscious of our existence and joy. All that has been has lead to our current condition of being. How we orchestrate our present state of being will influence the development of the future. It means that all experiences are remembered and saved in the 26 (like in a hard-drive) and already contain the tracks for future events. Therefore be aware of the now!

The 26 has the sum 8, which means rhythm, peace and strength. The 8 consists of 2 circles that are connected to each other as man combines heaven and earth in himself.

The 26 is the higher frequency of 8 with the experiences of all energy locks and the ability of foresight to oversee everything like a good director.

Support / Assistance:
- Lack of vitality
- Stubbornness
- Congestion, tumours and other accumulations
- Complete harmony of being (not only to exist)

Practice:
- Hold each finger
- Put palms together as in praying

- 🖐 R   left 26

    🖐 L   right 24

- 🖐 R   left 26

    🖐 L   left 15

- 🖐 R   left 24

    🖐 L   right 26

- 🖐 R   right 15

    🖐 L   right 26

The Organ Flows

As we have learned, the main central flow connects us with the universal energy and nourishes us and our organs every moment of life. It is our energy supplier and should be maintained regularly with care so that it flows abundantly through us and makes us feel to be in the flow of life. From there emerge the 12 organ flows; they are like little excursions of the central flow, supply the particular body areas and specifically one organ which gives its name to this particular part of the energy. Organ and energy flow are one unit. All organ flows merge with the main central flow and with many unmentioned energy flows that compose the complete energy cycle.

Every two hours another organ flow takes over the leadership.

At four o'clock in the morning the day begins with the lung energy, the lung flow. It has the support of the entire system but also the burden of leadership. At six o'clock the large intestine energy takes over and the lung energy goes to the back of the line. The following describes the flows by their temporal order. Thus, it is easy to understand that no body part and no energy section can be treated separately without influencing the entire circulation. Each body organ has its specific task within the body's community. This is reflected in certain body areas and can be influenced by our thoughts and actions, through our attitude and our awareness.

This shows that changes in the body are always and at any time possible when the energy flow pulses through us and we become the flowing energy.

If an organ needs special attention, we can then lead and support the flow with our hands. Each organ flow has its own predetermined task corresponding to the combination of the touched energy locks. Each of the twelve organ flows is related to a sign of the zodiac and therefore defined by it, for example the lung flow with its sign 'Aries' has the quality 'I am'. The meaning of the individual energy locks we are touching helps this quality to develop. Both, a right and a left flow are specified. You decide spontaneously which one to harmonize. No need to do both because they communicate with each other. Of course you can do both if you wish. As noted, move the hands step by step, with one hand remaining in its place while the other wanders.

In case you lack time, only hold the first step of the equivalent organ flow, known as 'anchor step', because it gives the healing direction.

The Lungs

The lungs are astrologically associated with Aries and the lung flow says: '**I am**'.

The lung's energy unfolds at birth, with the first cry, likewise each day early in the morning the lung supplies us with energy and power. With our breath, the lung-energy forms the basis of our personality, which is expressed as 'I am'. This strengthens the confidence and self awareness in our exchange with the environment and other people. Our contact and ability to communicate often show in the condition of our skin, which is a mirror of our inner life – 'as inside so outside'. Lung-energy strengthens the immune system and allows an age-appropriate development and the formation of common sense together with a good mental and spiritual constitution.

Harmonize your lungs by holding the ring fingers or practice the lung flow in a meditative context.

Support / Assistance:
- Sadness
- Weak lungs, cough, hoarseness
- Cold, flu, breathing difficulties
- Skin disease, acne, eczema, neurodermatitis
- Immune system
- Feeling of guilt

Lung Flow

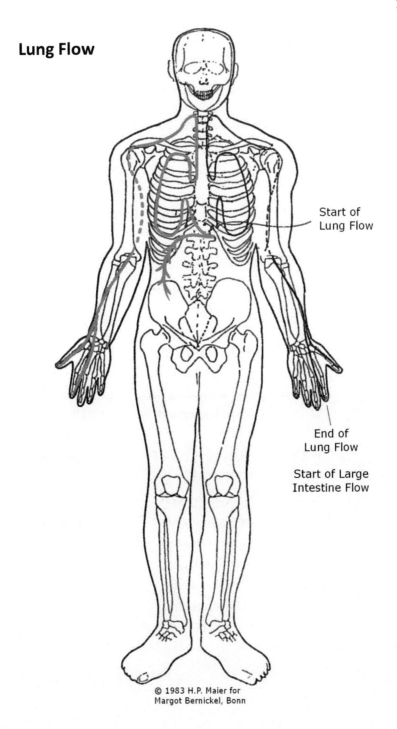

Start of
Lung Flow

End of
Lung Flow

Start of Large
Intestine Flow

© 1983 H.P. Maier for
Margot Bernickel, Bonn

Lung Flow (Energy Function)

04:00 – Aries – 'I am'

	Left flow			Right flow
1.	left 22	My will and my balance,		left 14
	right 14	nourished through all elements and the 144,000 body functions, help to perceive, how I am,		right 22
2.	left high 19	take and bring me into leadership,		right high 19
3.	left 18	development of body consciousness		right 18
4.	left 11	to recognize my excess baggage and to let go,		right 11
5.	right 22	experiencing the abundance of energy		left 22

6. right 13   to use it for me   left 13
                                      and also
                                      for others.
                                 That way I know,
                                   that 'I am'.

The Large Intestine - Colon

The colon is astrologically associated with the Bull and says: **'I have'**.

There we have the dilemma: The Bull is the concept of pleasure and stored food. The duty of the colon is to absorb and give away (excrete) in equal parts. The human being remains constantly in this interplay between receiving and releasing. This principle is always valid for both physical and mental possessions: experience, process, release and create space for the new. Sometimes this process, in the intestines and in the mind, takes time. Analogue to the intestines, the intensive study of a subject, usually leads to a firm or even fixed opinion, which will be strongly or even stubbornly maintained with the motto: 'I found out' (constipation).

To let go of one's own opinion, leaving a solid soil or the passive suffering of a loss leads to uncertainty and sadness.

Harmonize your colon by holding the ring finger or practice the large intestine flow in a meditative way.

Support / Assistance:
- Constipation, abdominal pain
- Diarrhoea
- Skin irritations
- Emotional tension
- Teeth aches, bleeding gums
- Neuralgia
- Throat pain / inflammation

Large Intestine Flow

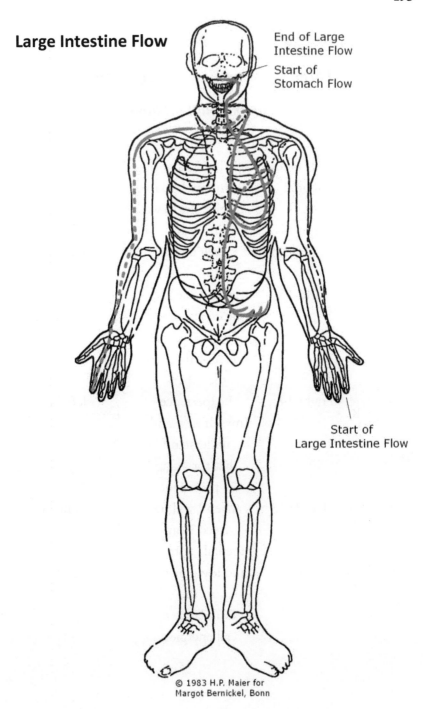

End of Large
Intestine Flow

Start of
Stomach Flow

Start of
Large Intestine Flow

Large Intestine Flow (Energy Function)

06:00 - Bull – 'I have'

	Left flow			*Right flow*	
1.	R	left index finger	What I have I learn to let go to receive the new.	R	left 11
	L	right 11	My fears melt away	L	right index finger
2.	R	right 13	and let me see the creation, my divine essence and also those in the others	L	left 13
3.	R	right 14	I experience myself new and understand that for living is provided,	L	left 14
4.	R	left 21	when I will be freed from mental captivity	L	right 21
5.	R	right 22	and leave myself to the abundance of all energies	L	left 22

6. left 22   and thus have   right 22

the freedom and

abundance.

The Stomach

The stomach is astrologically associated with Gemini and says: '**I think**'.

Of all things, the stomach, of which we expect the earthly task of practical food processing, says: 'I think'. The stomach is precisely the aspect of man that connects practical work with the ability to think. The stomach flow starts its path at 21, the energy lock of spiritual liberation. From there it ascends, frees the mind and thoughts and protects us from gloomy, depressive thoughts. It also acts like a plastic surgeon as it strengthens the lymphatic flow, gives clear skin and helps us to digest material and spiritual matter.

Harmonize your stomach with the thumb or practice the stomach flow in a meditative way.

Support / Assistance:
- Digestion
- Belching, tooth ache
- Heavy legs and arms
- Stuffy nose
- Dry mouth, brittle lips
- Concern, worries, grief, brooding

Stomach Flow

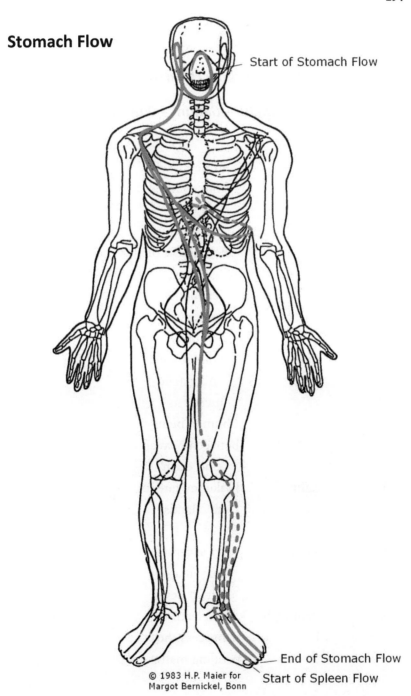

Start of Stomach Flow

End of Stomach Flow
Start of Spleen Flow

© 1983 H.P. Maier for
Margot Bernickel, Bonn

Stomach Flow (Energy Function)

08.00 – Gemini – 'I think'

	Left flow			*Right flow*	
1.	R	left 21	I free myself from spiritual captivity	R	right 22
	L	left 22	and receive the fullness of energy, elements, colours and sounds.	L	right 21
2.	L	right 14	I digest and understand myself as a human being between heaven and earth	R	left 14
3.	L	right 23	I take my fate in my hands.	R	left 23
4.	L	left 14	I accept myself as a human being	R	right 14
5.	L	right high 1	and learn to process the pending matters	R	left high 1

6. right deep 8   to see them in the context of the rhythmic double arc   left deep 8

7. right middle toe   and bring them through myself to the ground.   left middle toe

The Spleen

The spleen is astrologically associated with Cancer and says: **'I feel'.**

In Eastern medicine, the spleen has a very high priority. It is the organ of the solar plexus, because it gathers and keeps the sun energy to pass it to the other organs. It also strengthens the immune, lymphatic and nervous systems. As an organ with its ascending energy it supplies us with ground forces and stabilizes our defences against viruses, bacteria and fungi. Via the spleen flow we obtain basic trust to accept responsibility for ourselves and our lives.

We no longer need to chase after 'missed opportunities', but can get along with ourselves very well.

Harmonize the spleen with the thumbs or practice the spleen flow in a meditative way.

Support / Assistance:
- Digestion, flatulence
- Nervous system
- Heaviness in body
- Weight gain, cellulite
- Weakness of connective tissue
- Fatigue, lack of energy
- Craving for sweets
- Brooding
- Being grounded

Spleen Flow

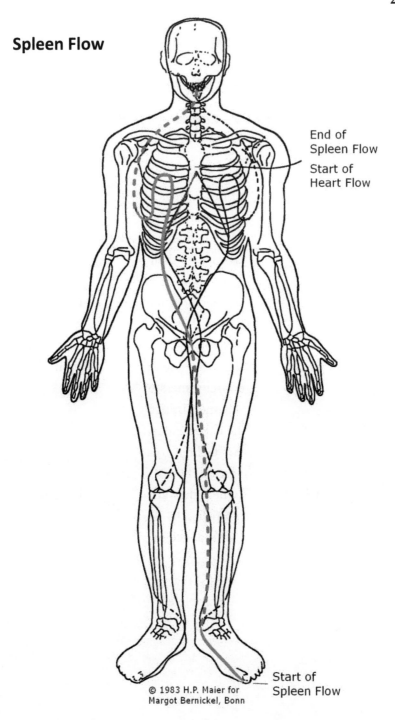

End of
Spleen Flow

Start of
Heart Flow

Start of
Spleen Flow

Spleen Flow (Energy Function)

10.00 – Cancer – 'I feel'

Left flow		Right flow	
1. R coccyx	Becoming aware of my feelings as a human being	R right 5	
L left 5	I gradually recognize their roots	L coccyx	
2. L right 14	as they hold me when I am in unstable balance.	R left 14	
3. R left 13	The dawning of consciousness of creation brings the experience of my feelings to a greater height,	L right 13	
4. R right 22	where they are nourished by the abundance of energy, so that I may feel complete.	L left 22	

The Heart

The heart is astrologically associated with Lion and says: **'I want to'**.

Ernst Schönwiese said: *"What beats in your heart so powerfully, is the person who you really are, let him go."*

The heart has a central position as the most powerful organ, which comes first and goes last and also as a symbol and embodiment of life and love. The heart is the synonym for love on each level, whether physically, materially, emotionally or religiously. In our bodies the heart works as an engine, and sends the blood untiringly through arteries and veins.

The heart is a muscle that should be treated very well. Therefore caution should be exercised in extreme fasting; it makes muscle tissue break down, including the heart.

All our emotions are registered by the heart and answered with an appropriate heartbeat.

Therefore a changed heart beat can have many reasons like psychological causes, weather conditions or heavy meals, but also serious medical reasons.

Before getting medical clarification, harmonize your heart with the little fingers, or practice the heart flow with the meditative sense.

Mary Burmeister said: *"Be patient to all unsolved matters in your heart."*

Support / Assistance:
* Tightness of the heart area, radiating to the upper arms
* Feverish palms
* Language difficulties, mental confusion

- Nerves, depression
- Excessive adjustment (pretending)

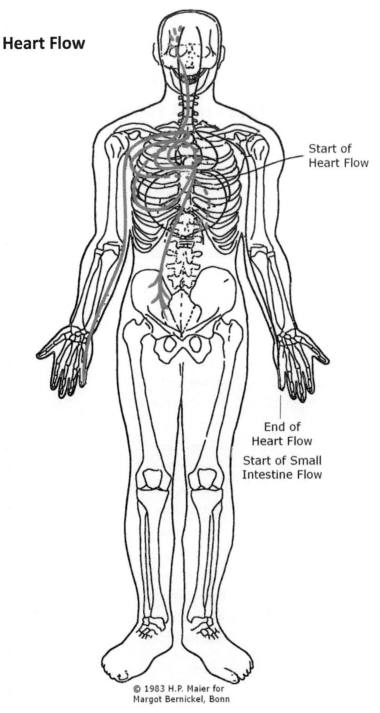

Heart Flow

Start of
Heart Flow

End of
Heart Flow

Start of Small
Intestine Flow

© 1983 H.P. Maier for
Margot Bernickel, Bonn

Heart Flow (Energy Function)

12:00 – Lion – 'I want to'

Left flow			Right flow	
1.	R — left 17	I want to rid myself of excess baggage and am the 'dropping' of my shoulders,	R — right 11	
	L — left 11	my nerves and my mind clean themselves, so that my heart can take over the lead.	L — right 17	
2.	R — right 22	The abundance of my energy flows freely, distributes elements, sounds and colours in me so that I	L — left 22	
3.	R — right 14	myself experience the here and now,	L — left 14	
4.	R — right 15	with laughter, joy and harmony,	L — left 15	

5.   R   left 1   stride forward in   L   right 1
my wholeness,

6.   R   left 5   experience my   L   right 5
5 senses as a
human being

7.   R   left 7   and swing myself   L   right 7
victoriously
over them,
as I want to.

The Small Intestine

The small intestine is astrologically associated with Virgo and says: '**I analyze**'.

The main task of the small intestine is to analyze, digest and distribute the transformed food to body and mind, as well as to prepare the immune system. But hardly anyone talks about the small intestine. It works incognito and in secret, however, precise and reliable, similar to a Virgo-born surgeon who works mostly unrecognized.

Likewise, many diseases of the small intestine are difficult to diagnose and therefore remain undetected. It is indeed very sensitive without complaining noticeably, but suffers in silence.

Harmonize your small intestine by holding the little fingers or practice the small intestine flow in a meditative way.

Support / Assistance:
- Diarrhoea, flatulence, digestion
- Sore throat, flu
- Ear aches
- Sinus problems
- Stiff neck, aching shoulders
- Tooth ache
- Compulsiveness, fussiness

Small Intestine Flow

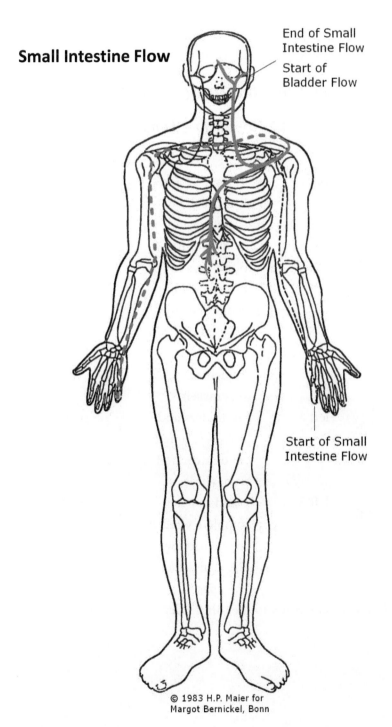

End of Small
Intestine Flow

Start of
Bladder Flow

Start of Small
Intestine Flow

Small Intestine Flow (Energy Function)

14:00 – Virgo – 'I analyze'

Left flow			*Right flow*	
1. (R)	right 13	I analyze and recheck my nature and	(R)	right 11
(L)	left 11	consign myself to the laws of the creator with his renewal energy, and	(L)	left 13
2. (R)	right 19*	learn to implement it on myself,	(L)	left 19*
3. (R)	left 1	to understand myself as a new and integrated whole,	(L)	right 1
4. (R)	left 7	and to reach complete vitality: my victory over the analysis and myself.	(L)	right 7

* For self-help, reach to the other side.

The Bladder

The bladder is astrologically associated with Libra and says: **'We balance'**.

The bladder speaks in plural because to the right and left of the spine, there are three descending energy paths. That means they flow in the opposite direction of the main central flow. It is easy to imagine that an interference of these flows can happen, especially when in fear, pain or cramps. This leads to a crooked posture causing a disturbed flow.

A blocked bladder flow with its pathways at the back can often cause back pain and pressure in the head. Libra born people may suffer from bladder issues and are hesitant in deciding.

Harmonize your bladder with the index fingers and practice the bladder flow in a meditative way.

Support / Assistance:
- Weak bladder, bed wetting
- Fear, phobia
- Back pain, muscle cramps, aching bones and joints
- Head pressure, dizziness, ringing in the ears

Bladder Flow

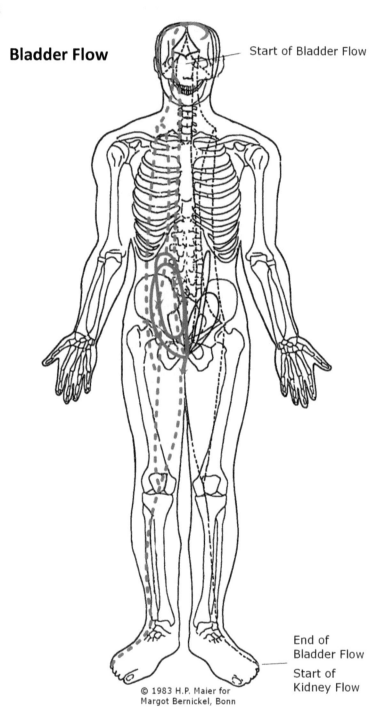

Start of Bladder Flow

End of
Bladder Flow

Start of
Kidney Flow

Bladder Flow (Energy Function)

16:00 – Libra – 'We balance'

Left flow			Right flow	
1.	left 25	The devotion to the will of the Creator		right 12
	left 12	will allow my regeneration in silence		right 25
2.	left back of knee	and helps me in moving forward,		right back of knee
3.	left 16	checks the basics of all my actions,		right 16
4.	left 23	helps me to take my fate in my own hands and		right 23
5.	left 9*	helps me to complete and to get rid of old patterns,		right 9*
6.	left 10*	to start new with the abundance of experience		right 10*

7. left 3 and to be in Right 3
harmony and in
perfect balance.

* Omit step 5 and 6 when practicing self-help.

The Kidneys

The kidneys are astrologically associated with Scorpio and say: '**I renew**'.

From birth, the kidneys supply our root energy for all organs and therefore embody our life's essence. Their main task is to filter blood and the production of urine which contains excreted substances. The kidneys 'thoroughly analyze the blood' and continuously renew this essential body fluid, like the Scorpio constantly questions the status quo and tries to look 'behind the curtain'. For their work, the kidneys need sufficient fluid. The kidneys' energy function helps us to reduce deep-seated fear, guilt complex, feelings of inferiority and to learn self-love.

Harmonize the kidneys with the index fingers or practice the kidney flow in a meditative way.

Support / Assistance:
- Circulation, blood pressure, blood cleansing
- Feeling cold, poor circulation
- Vein problems
- Ears, equilibrium
- Reproductive organs, sexuality
- Fears, self-esteem
- Addiction

Kidney Flow

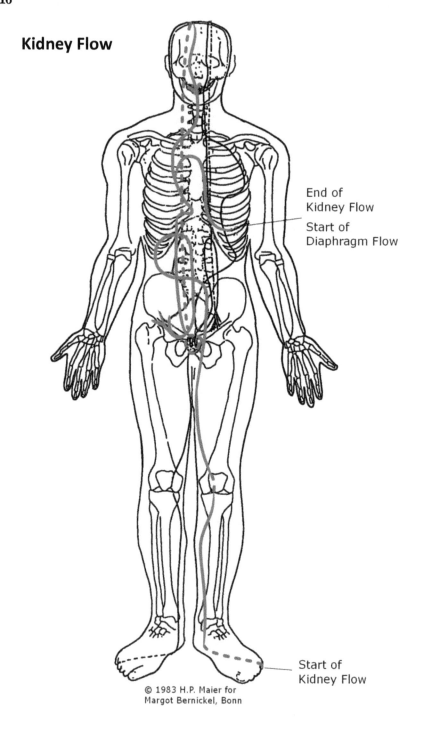

End of
Kidney Flow

Start of
Diaphragm Flow

Start of
Kidney Flow

© 1983 H.P. Maier for
Margot Bernickel, Bonn

Kidney Flow (Energy Function)

18:00 – Scorpio – 'I create' – 'I renew'

	Left flow			Right flow
1.	R — left little toe	The primal forces of renewal mix	R — pubic bone	
	L — pubic bone	with the root energy	L — right little toe	
2.	R — coccyx	and the earth energy.	L — coccyx	
3.	L — right 14	I check myself and my current status in the world where I am	R — left 14	
4.	L — right 13	and put myself in relation to the creative power	R — left 13	
5.	L — right 12	and to the will of the Creator, so that I can renew my point of view.	R — left 12	

The Diaphragm

The diaphragm is astrologically associated with Sagittarius and says: '**I recognize, I perceive**'.

Sagittarius, with an arrow and bow, concentrates on the target that he perceives and recognizes with a keen eye. The art of archery teaches to merge with the target till the arrow is released and meets the true target.

The focus on the distant target is, at the same time, a look within. This aspect of unification reflects the diaphragm and is considered to be a source of life. Its dome-shaped partition of the chest and abdomen plays an important role in the breath, our great healer.

Harmonize your diaphragm with your palms or practice the diaphragm flow in a meditative way.

Support / Assistance:
- Respiration
- Protection for all organs
- Tension in elbows, hips, waist, thighs
- Night visibility
- Heart pressure via the so called elevated diaphragm
- Extroversion
- Nightmares, sleeping problems

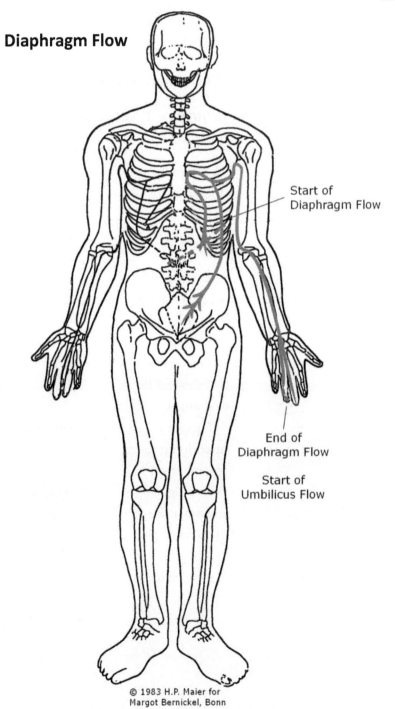

Diaphragm Flow

Start of
Diaphragm Flow

End of
Diaphragm Flow

Start of
Umbilicus Flow

Diaphragm Flow (Energy Function)

20:00 - Sagittarius – 'I recognize'

	Left flow			Right flow	
1.	R	right 19*	I recognize myself in my being as I am,	R	right 14
	L	left 14	in my authority and responsibility,	L	left 19*
2.	L	left 25	I become tranquil and experience renewal	R	right 25
3.	R	right 5	as I reconsider my fears and let them go.	L	left 5
4.	R	right palm	I lead my attention into my inner-self	L	left palm
5.	R	left ring finger	and recognize my inner fire, which feeds and leads me.	L	right ring finger

* For self-help, reach to the other side.

The Umbilicus

The umbilicus is astrologically associated with Capricorn and says: '**I use**'.

The separation from the umbilical cord at birth is the navel, our first elemental scar. Externally apart, we remain invisibly connected to the cosmic energy which is available to us in abundance.

Each scar contains all information and power that lead to it. Therefore it can contribute to our understanding if we search for this power. Thus, the navel energy is also responsible for access and connections since a Capricorn remains grounded despite the lofty heights.

To harmonize your umbilicus hold your palms or practice the umbilicus flow in a meditative way.

Support / Assistance:

- Thermal regulation
- Absorption and excretion
- Shaping the body
- Ear problems
- Distribution in the body and mediation
- Fatigue issues
- Process of independence

Umbilical Flow

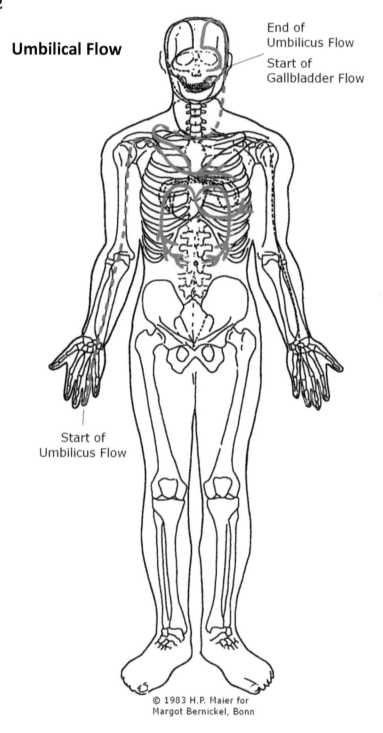

End of
Umbilicus Flow

Start of
Gallbladder Flow

Start of
Umbilicus Flow

© 1983 H.P. Maier for
Margot Bernickel, Bonn

Umbilical Flow (Energy Function)

22:00 – Capricorn – 'I use'

Left flow			Right flow	
1.	left 19	I need my clear vision or the clearing of the vision		left 20
	right 20	to recognize my true authority		right 19
2.	right 12	and place it under 'thy sake'		left 12
3.	right 14	to come		left 14
4.	left 14	to myself,		right 14
5.	right 23	to accept my fate,		left 23
6.	right 25	to regenerate at rest,		left 25

7. right 16   to rethink the left 16
source of my
activities

8. right ring   and to create   left ring
finger   new elixir or life   finger
for my
personal use.

The Gallbladder

The gallbladder is astrologically associated with Aquarius and says: '**I know**'.

The bile is a very important secretion of the liver, which in concentrated form is stored in the gall bladder, especially for fat digestion. Since bile is continuously produced in the liver, it should be used for food digestion to prevent an overflow of the gall and not to 'spit poison and gall' nor produce gall stones. Excessive rage, anger, envy, frustration and even suppressed emotions burden the function of the gall-bladder, which can lead to congestion, often experienced as headaches, migraines and pain in the lumbar area.

If you want to calm down, moderately enforce your intentions by holding your middle fingers or practice the gall bladder flow in a meditative way.

Support / Assistance:
- Bitter taste, burping, bloating
- Pain in back and pelvic area
- Lumbago, sciatica
- Lateral head ache, migraine
- Stiff neck, draught-sensitive, gout
- Nightmares, deep sighs
- Fat-intolerance, digestion problems
- Shivers
- View and mental clarity

Gallbladder Flow

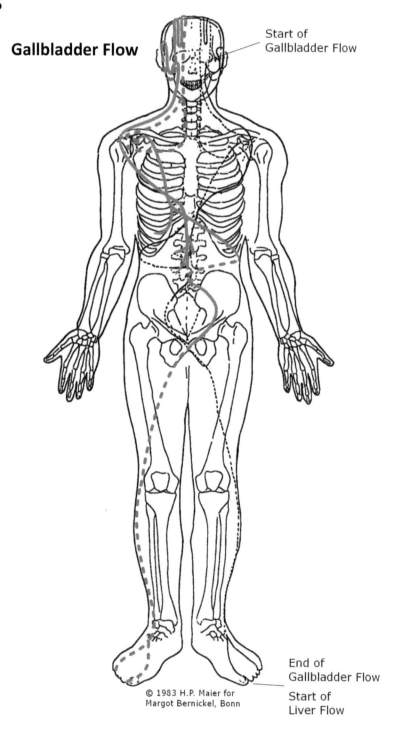

Start of
Gallbladder Flow

End of
Gallbladder Flow

Start of
Liver Flow

© 1983 H.P. Maier for
Margot Bernickel, Bonn

Gallbladder Flow (Energy Function)

24:00 – Aquarius – 'I know'

Left flow			Right flow	
1.	right 20	I know that 'Your will'		right 12
	left 12	opens my eyes for other dimensions,		left 20
2.	coccyx	I realize where my source is,		coccyx
3.	right 16	where my bases for my being are		left 16
4.	right 14	and how I can bring them		left 14
5.	left 14	here into this world		right 14
6.	left 22	and I know of all this abundance with all the elements, colour, sound and all the energy.		right 22

The Liver

The liver is astrologically associated with Pisces and says: **'I believe'**.

In the past the location of the liver had been associated with the centre of life, which is obvious to point out the importance of its task. As the largest gland and detoxification station of the body, the liver has a very central role for the entire metabolism. It has its peak at night, in which it quietly cleanses the blood and prepares for the new day. Only after a very long period of strain it demands absolute care for it becomes irritated, annoyed and even disgusted with certain foods.

With the liver flow, body, mind and spirit come back into balance before the new day begins with the lung flow.

Harmonize your liver with the middle fingers or practice the liver flow in a meditative way.

Support / Assistance:
- Headaches behind the eyes, migraine
- Itchy eyes, red eyes
- Hay fever
- Brittle, torn nails
- Exhaustion
- Joint pain, gout, tendons, spine
- Prejudice, stubbornness, choleric personality

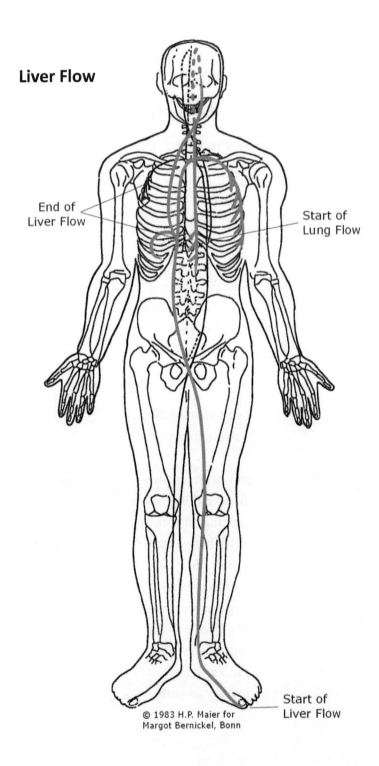

Liver Flow

End of
Liver Flow

Start of
Lung Flow

Start of
Liver Flow

© 1983 H.P. Maier for
Margot Bernickel, Bonn

Liver Flow (Energy Function)

02:00 – Pisces – 'I believe'

	Left flow			Right flow	
1.	R	right 22	I believe in the connection between mind / spirit	R	right 4
	L	left 4	and the elements as well as all forms of energy.	L	left 22
2.	R	right 14	They feed me,	L	left 14
3.	R	left 1	so I can boldly stride forward	L	right 1
4.	R	left 5	and overcome my fears and human entanglements.	L	right 5
5.	R	left 18	With help of the new physical consciousness	L	right 18
6.	L	right 4	I experience myself as a bridge to the spiritual world: faith as reality or reality as faith.	R	left 4

Important First Aid

Critical situations usually trigger a shock to the individual involved as well as for those who are present. Sometimes there is not enough time left to look at the appropriate Jin Shin Jyutsu steps before the doctor comes.

Therefore some important short steps:
- **Seizure, confusion:**
  Hold both 4, then both 7
  Or: One person holds the 4 the other the 7
- **Bleeding:**
  Hold right hand on it, the left hand cross wise above (possibly floating)
- **Angina:**
  Hold both wrists
- **Convulsions:**
  Hold mid 23
- **Fainting:**
  Hold both 4
- **Accident, surgery, critical situation:**
  Finger-toe-flow, (see p. 64)
- **Burns:**
  Left hand floating above, right hand on top
- **Swallowed down the wrong pipe:**
  Hold both high 1 cross wise

Further Information

For further information please take a look at the following websites:
www.jin-shin-fee.de – my website (German)
www.jinshinjyutsu.creative-story.de – my blog (English)

You can contact me:
via e-mail at: graefinwaldeck@creative-story.com
or send me a fax to: +49 (0) 89 / 930 19 16

Thanks

To Mary Burmeister and her teacher Jiro Murai and her students who became teachers. Thanks for spreading the knowledge of Jin Shin Jyutsu into so many hearts.

I thank my patients and my friends for the possibility of transformation and the many wonderful experiences with them.

Many thanks especially to Ingrid Sassner who had the idea of translating this book into English, which she did with amazing patience, enthusiasm and loving energy.

Also many thanks to Monika Schulze, Art Neeland and Regina Puga-Hertzsch, who corrected the English version.

Special thanks to Roswitha Gerhart, who had the idea to transform this book into an eBook so that this wonderful Human-Creator-Art Jin Shin Jyutsu can be more easily reached by a wide audience spanning all age groups.

Illustrations

Legend:

   Flow at the backside

   Flow at the body front

Index

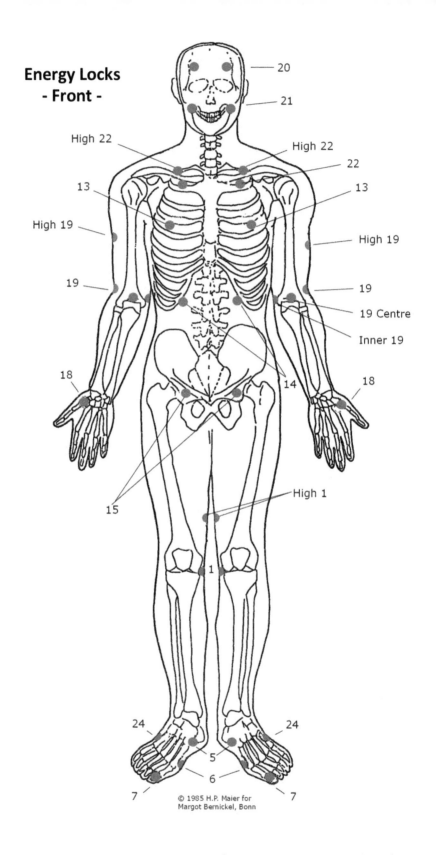

Energy Locks
- Front -

20

21

High 22

High 22

22

13

13

High 19

High 19

19

19

19 Centre

Inner 19

18

18

14

15

High 1

1

24

24

5

6

7

7

© 1985 H.P. Maier for
Margot Bernickel, Bonn

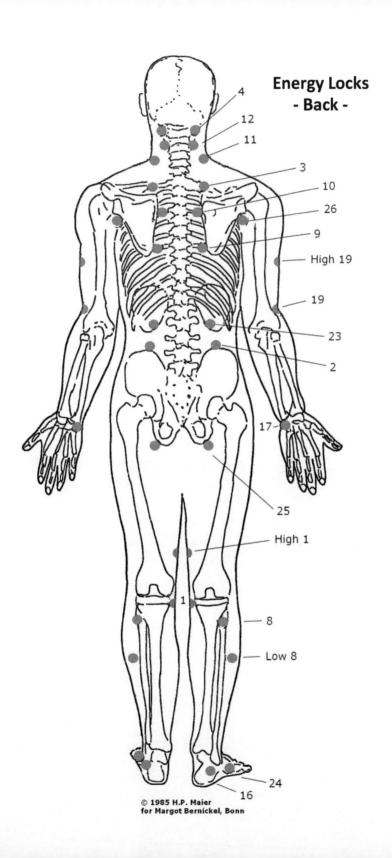

Energy Locks
- Back -

4
12
11
3
10
26
9
High 19
19
23
2
17
25
High 1
1
8
Low 8
24
16

© 1985 H.P. Maier
for Margot Bernickel, Bonn

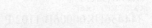

Lightning Source UK Ltd.
Milton Keynes UK
UKHW021123150619
344456UK00006B/1102/P